THE
Medical
Elite

T0320954

THE
Medical
Elite
Training for
Leadership

Stephen J. Miller

With a foreword by
Everett C. Hughes

ALDINETRANSACTION
A Division of Transaction Publishers
New Brunswick (U.S.A.) and London (U.K.)

First paperback printing 2011 by Transaction Publishers, New Brunswick, NJ
Copyright © 1970 by Transaction Publishers, New Brunswick, NJ

This book is printed on acid-free paper that meets the American National
Standard for Permanence of Paper for Printed Library Materials.

Library of Congress Catalog Number: 2010020491
ISBN 978-0-202-36358-5
Printed in the United States of America

Library of Congress Cataloging-in-Publication Data

Miller, Stephen J.
    [Prescription for leadership]
    The medical elite : training for leadership / Stephen J. Miller ; with a
    foreword by Everett C. Hughes. -- New paperback ed.
        p. ; cm.
    Originally published as: Prescription for leadership / Stephen J. Miller.
    Chicago : Aldine Pub., 1970.
    Includes index.
    ISBN 978-0-202-36358-5 (pbk. : alk. paper)
        1. Interns (Medicine)--Massachussetts--Boston. 2. Boston City Hospital.
    Harvard Medical Unit I. Title. [DNLM: 1. Boston City Hospital. Harvard Medical
    Unit. 2. Hospitals. 3. Internship and Residency. 4. Internal Medicine--education.
    5. Leadership. 6. Organizational Case Studies. WX 203 M651m 1970a]

R840.M54 2010
610.71'174461--dc22
                                                                    2010020491

Acknowledgments

MANY FRIENDS and colleagues have offered valuable advice and assistance in the preparation of this manuscript, but there is no way to acknowledge them all individually. There is also no way to determine the value of suggestions or insights of colleagues who took the time to listen and responded to ideas. I am, of course, greatly indebted to my colleagues at Brandeis University.

A few people were particularly helpful. I am most indebted to Blanche Geer, who took the time to meet regularly with me and provided invaluable ideas, insights, and criticisms that improved the study. Without her continued assistance, I would have been unable to complete the study. My efforts were also encouraged by Howard S. Becker and Everett C. Hughes. I am grateful for their encouragement and am indebted to them for improving that part of my work that is sociology. I am also grateful for the friendship of Howard E. Freeman, who supported my efforts although he had a somewhat different sociological perspective. Finally I am indebted to Charles I. Schottland for his efforts on my behalf and his support of the study.

My thanks also to Osler Peterson and Charles S. Davidson of the Harvard Medical School. I am grateful to them for criticism that raised important questions regarding the issues with which the study deals. They were always available and willing to help. I am also grateful to Paul Sanazaro for encouraging my interest in medical education. He arranged opportunities for me to gain additional insights into the medical world. What is reported herein is based on research supported by the Cooperative Research Program of the Office of Education, U.S. Department of Health, Education and Welfare. I am grateful for that financial support and the additional assistance of its staff on matters relating to the study. The help of these people improved every page of this book, but they cannot be held responsible for my interpretation of what I observed at the Boston City Hospital.

The book has also been improved by the criticism of Robert H. Ebert. I am grateful for the time he took to read and discuss the manuscript, though I did not always agree with what he had to say. I also did not always agree with other physicians, but my encounters with them and their honest opinions improved my understanding of the medical elite. I am grateful for the interest and support of many physicians who may have considered me a critic but not an enemy.

I must also acknowledge the influence of Arnold M. Rose. His excellent counsel and sympathetic criticism of all my efforts have improved all that I have tried to do. My debt is acknowledged but not paid.

There is no way to adequately acknowledge the patience and tolerance of my wife, Roberta. I can only say that I appreciate all she has done for me and Andrew, Rodney, and Jessica during the many hours I spent away from home.

Finally, I appreciate the good humor and assistance of the interns with whom I spent my time in the field. The fact that they had a great deal of work to do never prevented them from participating in the study. A few will join the staff of the Center for Community Health and Medical Care at Harvard, and I will thank them personally. I want the other interns to know that I realize how generous they were, and I appreciate all that they did for me. For that reason, this book is not only about but for the interns of the Harvard Medical Services at the Boston City Hospital.

Foreword

THE MEDICAL profession is perhaps a community within a larger society, as William J. Goode likes to say. When people of any modern industrial society are asked to rate occupations, the physician comes, like cream, to the top. It is indeed true that nearly all younger physicians have run a course of schooling that is identical in many respects; twelve years of pre-collegiate education, four years of college, four years of medical school. In the clinical years of their medical course, they will have gone behind the medical counter to help serve the laymen. But not even at the end, when they are dubbed Doctors of Medicine, are they full members of the community of which Goode speaks. Before them lies the internship and, very likely, a residency in some specialty. At the last moment before internship, the "almost physicians" may be more nearly a homogeneous group than they will ever be again.

The internships and residencies that make sure and deepen their membership in the medical community make the young physicians different from each other; different not only in kind and degree of skill, but also in their concepts and philosophy of health and disease, and of their own roles and careers in an ever more complicated medical system. Interns and residents come to be more closely associated with some breeds of doctors than with others. Some get badges of identity; "He is one of Dr.———'s men," or "he was trained in———hospital."

This book reports the course of a group of medical college graduates through their internship in internal medicine in a Boston City Hospital; this is an internship directed by a full-time member of the staff of the prestigeful Harvard Medical School. Although many hospitals cannot attract their full quota of interns, the Boston City internship is much sought after. The building is a miserable affair, fit to be condemned. The patients come in—or are brought in—off the streets. They are not the patients that would attract others and thus form the nucleus of a good, middle-class clientele; they have neither money nor influence. The building and the patients are at the bottom of the heap, but the internship is at the top. How can that be? Because every intern comes knowing that much is expected of him, that no excuses can be made for failure to live up to the expectation, and that he is in the anteroom to the club of successful medical men.

What the interns don't know is how hard they will have to work (although all medical students work hard), and they don't really know what the expectations are; least of all do they know the nature of the human organization they must learn to operate to get their work done. Their daily labor consists of dozens of social transactions, mostly small. The interns have little weight of authority to throw around. They must make their bargains in economy of exchanges without money or other material rewards or sanctions. They can't even "get anyone's job." To do their work they must get reciprocating action from many other people. It is perhaps the ideal type of the situation where one must learn—learn socially—to survive. But if one does survive, the potential rewards are great, and that is what distinguishes this situation from many others.

The young physician who comes to the United States from a

poor country to do an internship or residency may work in a hospital physically superior to Boston City, but he may not be in a position to win any of his contests with others in the system. He may not be able to call on distinguished "consults" to help him with diagnoses and treatment. He may, in fact, be a kind of doctor's-helper to the patients' private physician. Finally, he may know that if he returns to his native country he will never again have facilities equal to those he has as a resident in this country. That is another learning situation; probably not a good one.

To understand how medical students grow into the many different kinds of physicians at work in our sickness-and-health system, we need to work out the variables of the situations in which they make the transition from student to practitioner and in which the identification with a style of practice and a close group of colleagues takes place. Then we must study these various settings as Stephen Miller has studied this one so that valid comparisons can be made. To complete such a program of study and make it useful, the later careers of people who have learned their professions in various settings must be looked at. Even good men deteriorate in certain circumstances.

Viewed in one way, a profession is an occupation about which people have strong and perhaps idealized conceptions before they enter training. The training is long; acceptance as a full colleague comes late. At some point in the training, and before full acceptance, the aspirant is put to work in some institution where he or she begins to learn by doing. This situation is the point of contact of universities and professional schools with the "real world."

In an era of increasing numbers of professions and of professional people, this point of contact of the academic world with the world of practice is "where the action is;" not with respect to medicine alone, but in many fields of social activity. Stephen Miller records and analyzes this action in a particular and crucial setting.

Everett C. Hughes

Contents

1. The Medical Elite—A Framework for the Study : 3
2. Problems and Proof of Observations : 17
3. The Harvard Unit at Boston City Hospital : 35
4. Candidates for the Medical Elite : 56
5. The Work of an Internship : 90
6. Learning the Work of an Internship : 117
7. Social Exchange and Dynamics of Work : 134
8. Perspectives on Work : 180
9. Is an Elite Internship Different? : 208
10. Conclusion : 227
   Appendix. The Performance of Harvard Interns on Part III of the National Boards : 247
   Index : 251

1. The Medical Elite—
A Framework for the Study

A SOCIETY like ours needs many services that only specially trained people can provide. More than ever we depend on highly skilled professionals; we delegate to them the responsibility for applying knowledge and we allow them to define for us matters pertaining to their work. The decisions and practices of one or another of the professions influence much of our way of living.

We often assume that all members of a profession are more or less alike. We think of a profession as a group of specialists who agree on their essential purpose—on what it is they should do for society. But unanimity is no more characteristic of professionals than of any other group of workers. While some accept one definition of their profession's purpose, others may feel that a different definition best serves society's needs.

Medicine, the most established of the professions, is no exception. Some physicians believe its purpose to be the scientific investigation of disease: they choose careers of teaching and research at hospitals or medical schools. Others think teaching and research less important than applying the knowledge we already have, and they choose careers of practice. In addition to this organizational division, specialties whose members organize their careers around particular aspects of medicine further divide the medical profession. This variety of opinion and careers produces subgroups whose members are more like one another than like members of other subgroups within medicine. Thus we see not one but many groups of physicians, each with a purpose and typical career of its own.

A professional career requires long years of training and study. During the training years, candidates for a profession learn its sciences and techniques, choose specific careers for themselves, and acquire the ideology of one of its several subgroups. An ideology distinguishes the relative value of the different kinds of work the profession claims as its own and describes the relation of careers organized around that particular work to other groups within the profession, other occupations, the public, and the institutions of society. When we attempt to understand the part a profession plays in our society, we must consider the processes by which its members are recruited, trained, and distributed among the subgroups that make decisions and change or maintain practices that affect us.

Sociologists interested in the professions have conducted many studies of medicine. My specific concern in this study is with one phase of the process by which candidates for the medical profession are recruited and trained and the implications of that recruitment and training for their subsequent careers in medicine. Although this is, in a sense, a study of medical education, I do not attempt to evaluate quality of training, but rather to describe and interpret sociologically a particular point in the progress of some young men toward careers in medicine: the experiences of interns at the Boston City Hospital, and the implications of that period of training for their future medical careers.

I observed medical school graduates serving internships at the Harvard Medical Unit of the Boston City Hospital, a place noted for training physicians for teaching and research. I was concerned with the processes by which young men are recruited and prepared for the first step on the ladder of an academic rather than of another kind of medical career.[1]

When the positions of a profession are defined in temporal relationship to one another, a career ladder exists within that profession. While the rungs of the career ladders of medical practice are not so obvious as, for example, those of the academic world, practicing physicians may be organized into distinct levels, each having increasing prerogatives and prestige. Together, they provide a career ladder to be climbed by the new member of the medical profession. A medical career begins with new members being admitted to positions of least responsibility and continues as they hold those positions or move on to different or higher positions in medicine.

Sociologists have often studied "successful" careers, observing how men entering at the bottom obtain positions of increasing responsibility and prestige that move them to the top of a profession. We know little, however, about why some men choose one rather than another kind of career, why some become academicians and others practitioners. We know even less about how they gain access to positions that begin those careers. My study suggests that individual medical careers result from processes occurring in medical schools and hospitals, which directly represent the social organization of the medical profession. It is these processes that will be examined here.

This implies some theory, or at least a rationale for interpreting observations. A particular sociological approach does serve as a framework for the study. Although I use most sociological concepts in the common way, a few differ from common usage. Some definitions are in order.

The concept of the professional elite requires some explanation. That concept evolved during my field work, as I tried to

1. Oswald Hall, "The Stages of a Medical Career," *American Journal of Sociology*, 53, 5 (March, 1948), pp. 327–336; also, "The Informal Organization of Medical Practice in an American City," a doctoral dissertation, University of Chicago, 1944.

explain the particular place of the Harvard Medical Unit in medicine and the implication of its existence for medical careers.

Some sociologists have assumed that professions are homogeneous work groups whose members agree on what their work should be and share interests, attitudes, and values that directly represent the purpose of their profession.[2] Others assume that professions are heterogeneous, encompassing not one but many work groups with the same occupational title.[3] Though an idealized career may symbolize the profession, as the general practitioner symbolizes medicine, each group controls careers organized around specific knowledge, particular skills, special interests, and unique purposes. Specialists are the most obvious examples of such a variety within a profession.

Although there are arguments for both approaches, an emphasis on homogeneity overlooks much of what we know about professions; it ignores, for example, the obvious differences among specialists and the conflict of interest between academicians and practitioners. I have therefore chosen the latter approach as the framework for my study.

A profession consists of a number of groups whose members attempt to obtain or maintain institutional positions that advance their special interests and facilitate the purpose of their group. These circles of colleagues share an identity and an ideology that lead them to organize their professional activity in similar ways. When referring to the organization of professions, I have in mind this phenomenon, the organization of which is determined by the activities and tactics of the segments.

The segments of a profession vary. Some are established segments whose claims have been recognized by the entire profession; their members have high status and usually hold institutional positions of power. Examples of established medical segments are internists, surgeons, and, in another profession, the psychiatric caseworker as opposed to the community organizer

2. For example, Robert K. Merton and others, *The Student Physician* (Cambridge, Harvard University Press, 1957).

3. Rue Bucher and Anselm Strauss, "Professions in Process," *American Journal of Sociology*, LXVI (January, 1961), pp. 325–334.

in social work. Other subgroups, not so well established, are still a recognized part of the profession (physical medicine, for example). Some segments are only emerging, like that of community psychiatry; they try to gain recognition and obtain appropriate positions for their members. At any particular period in the history of a profession these different kinds of groups are engaged in activities and tactics that will establish or entrench them further in the profession.

This view of professions as amalgamations of segments standing in some relationship to one another with respect to prestige and power leads us to consideration of the professional elite. "For every epoch and for every social structure," wrote Mills, "we must work out an answer to the question of the power of the elite." [4] Who are the elite within a profession? Why are they an elite? What is the basis of their status? Once established, how do they maintain their position?

At any given time in any profession, some segments have the most prestige and power, others have less, and some have little if any stature other than what they have as a part of the profession. To those segments with prestige and power we give the title "elite." [5]

When members of a segment obtain positions in the institutions of the profession, they acquire power. Power can be the right to make actual decisions determining the operations of an institution or influencing the practices of the profession or simply the right to participate in decision making. The latter form of power is, of course, limited, but participation affords members a voice in making decisions. Those professionals who actually make decisions will have additional power to implement

4. C. Wright Mills, *The Power Elite* (New York, Oxford University Press, 1957), p. 23.

5. Not all sociologists agree that those with power are the elite. Some, for example, Karl Mannheim, *Man and Society in an Age of Reconstruction,* argue that these are groups that have no power, or have not yet obtained power, but are influential in shaping a society. Others argue that differences in power are essential to making a distinction between the mass and the elite. See H. D. Lasswell and A. Kaplan, *Power and Society* (New Haven, Yale University Press, 1950). None, however, deny that power is an attribute of the elite.

them, but professionals who hold other positions can influence the decisions that are made and the ways in which they are implemented. Members of segments who obtain hold of institutional positions, therefore, have actual power or exercise a more subtle form of power.

Power, however, is not the only attribute of a professional elite. Today, the accumulated knowledge of any profession is so great that the members of any one segment cannot claim to know it all. They do, however, possess the knowledge relevant to the interests and purposes of their segment. Thus, in matters pertaining to its special interest, any one segment is intellectually superior to the other segments of the profession.

Power and intellectual superiority go hand in hand, and both are essential attributes of the established segments that constitute the elite of a profession. Without a recognized claim to intellectual superiority in a branch of the profession a segment would be denied power. On the other hand, segments with power can best maintain and enforce their claims to intellectual superiority. By so doing, they advance their interests and accomplish their purpose within the profession.

The professional elite, then, consists of members of segments with recognized claims to intellectual superiority who hold positions of power in the institutions of a profession. Each member of the elite owes his position to his relationship with a segment, and his activity gets its meaning for him and others from the avowed purpose of his segment. As a group, they are colleagues whose common interests and purpose lead them to wield power to guide the decisions and practices of their profession, supposedly for the good of all.

An elite so defined is not simply another segment. Segments may or may not have power. The elite always has power to influence the profession's decisions and practices. The membership of the elite may vary as circumstances undermine the claims of established segments and support those of emerging segments. Those segments that Bucher and Strauss refer to as "pockets of resistance and embattled minorities" are counterelites whose members may, in time, displace members of segments now included in the elite, making other decisions and affecting new practices.[6] The elite as a phenomenon, however, persists.

Two segments are common to almost all other divisions of the medical profession: the academic and the practicing. The academic segment, whose members have what may be called scientific interests, sees its primary purpose as the acquisition and communication of knowledge. Physicians at medical schools, regardless of specialty, belong to the academic segment of medicine. Members of the practice segment apply knowledge as a service. Since professions are founded on some esoteric knowledge, we might expect that those who excel at research and teaching would be set apart from the mass of those practicing the profession. A respect for scientific authority has justified the claims of some occupations to the title of "profession," and such respect could also serve among the scientifically trained to justify the existence of an elite.

I assume here, without providing proof, that members of the medical elite come from the academic segments, holding positions at teaching hospitals and medical schools. Others might argue that practitioners exert more influence. That argument overlooks significant facts about the organization of professions. Today, professions are rooted in institutions, and the policies and practices of those institutions are determined by men who occupy more or less permanent places in them. Practice usually refers to a private endeavor in, but not necessarily a part of, an institution.

Members of the medical elite stand on the career ladders of established segments. They have that status only so long as the segments they belong to have a reputation for superiority and control access to the career ladders of their branch of medicine. I have indicated why the reputation of the academic segment may be assumed to be greater than that of the practice segment of any branch of the profession. Moreover, the academic segment holds the best positions from which to control access to

6. Bucher and Strauss, "Professions in Process," p. 333.

career ladder positions at training institutions. Bucher and Strauss have noted the importance of these positions for segments:

> Segments are in competition for the allegiance of students: entire schools as well as single departments can be the arena of, and weapons in, this conflict [and] during their professional training, students pick their way through a maze of conflicting models and make momentous commitments thereby.[7]

Members of academic segments control the recruitment, socialization, and careers of physicians at the training institutions. When they recruit and train young men and women for careers that represent commitment to their own interests and purposes, they are also preparing new members for the medical elite.

The phrase "medical elite," to paraphrase Mills, refers to those circles of colleagues in which decisions are made that affect professions.[8] The members of this elite need not personally take part in every decision; they need only be among those whose opinions are taken seriously by persons making decisions.

As more and more professional activity is located in institutions, practitioners may make up more of the elite than they do now.[9] At present, however, the elite consists almost entirely of occupants of such institutional positions as researchers, teachers, and administrators. The elite of American medicine includes physicians occupying positions at "name" medical schools and hospitals that enable them to influence the teaching and the practice of medicine throughout the United States. I refer to "name" schools and hospitals in the sociological sense and imply no judgment of their quality. "Name" institutions need no further identification than the name: Harvard, Johns Hopkins, Columbia, Chicago, Pennsylvania, and a dozen or more schools generally accorded public esteem for the notable contributions of their scientists or the excellence of their teachers, students, and graduates. The public esteem for these schools makes them

---

7. Bucher and Strauss, "Professions in Process," p. 334.
8. C. Wright Mills, *The Power Elite*, p. 290.
9. There are examples of this happening in professions. For example, see Bucher, "Pathology: A Study of Social Movements Within a Profession," *Social Problems*, 1, 10 (Summer 1962), pp. 40–51.

the celebrities of American medicine, and the physicians at them are among the leaders of the medical elite.

At these medical schools and the hospitals affiliated with them (usually referred to as teaching hospitals), physicians are grouped by specialties into departments. Each department includes some practitioners, but the members of the academic segment far outnumber them, and they are the ones who decide matters pertaining to teaching, research, and administration. Since the academicians set the patterns for recruitment and socialization into the medical profession, they also define a route that candidates for academic careers must travel and decide the kinds of experiences they will have along the way.

All such routes consist of subordinate positions at schools and hospitals. A candidate seeking one rather than another medical career must travel a route of positions and experiences appropriate for that career. For academic careers, the route begins with the obtaining of a university-affiliated internship and continues through the "right" residency to teaching and research positions at medical schools and teaching hospitals.

When choosing internships, medical students know the routes that exist. Students who plan a traditional career worry only about obtaining internships that will provide them with practical experiences, preparing them for the general practice of medicine. They want internships at general hospitals. Those who plan to specialize know that the internship is but the first of several years of training, and that they must serve residencies of the right sort before they will be permitted careers of specialized practice. Almost any internship will do so long as it leads to an approved residency for the desired specialty. In contrast, students who include research and teaching in their future plans attach a great deal of importance to internships at university-affiliated hospitals, seeing this kind of internship as a necessary prelude to a residency that is "right" for a career dependent upon connections with medical schools and teaching hospitals.[10]

The candidates who follow these routes to academic careers

10. Howard S. Becker, Blanche Geer, Everett C. Hughes, and Anselm Strauss, *Boys in White* (Chicago, University of Chicago Press, 1961, pp. 384–400), discuss the choice of an intern in the way I have described.

have educational experiences of two kinds: (1) learning in the technical sense, acquiring knowledge and skill appropriate for a specialized practice; and (2) learning in the social sense, developing an identification with and commitment to a particular segment in a specialty of the medical profession. Some will climb the entire academic ladder and become members of the medical elite.

The Harvard Medical Unit is one of the segments that constitute the contemporary medical elite. My purpose is to understand the character of an elite segment and the implications of its activity for the experiences of young men preparing for medical careers. I therefore focus on the intern and attempt to understand his training in the light of Harvard activity at Boston City Hospital.

The training of physicians is, of course, only one of the objectives of a hospital. At most hospitals training is subservient to the primary objective of providing services to patients. Internships, in fact, enable hospitals to hire physicians to attend patients at little cost. Interns trade the time they spend attending patients for the experiences required of licensed physicians. An internship, then, resembles an apprenticeship: the organization not only trains people for medical careers, but also uses them to do essential work.

But internships also serve the purpose of the medical elite. The elite segments of medicine pay continued attention to the activity which earned them prestige and permitted them to accumulate power: They must continue to conduct medical research. As I show later, the internship is less an educational experience than it is a job. The job consists almost entirely of attending to patients; patients must be cared for if segments like the Harvard Medical Unit are to maintain themselves as hospitals and have access to patients for medical research. The Harvard Medical Unit has to provide that care. Internships, therefore, are a critical resource of the medical elite and a necessary condition for their existence at hospitals.

Interns are employees of the hospital and as such must do the work delegated to them, though doing so may reduce the educational value of their internship. What they have to do, for example, may have very little relation to what they will be doing in the future. Since the job must be done, however, interns spend the bulk of their time attending patients. They do so because it is the way to satisfactorily complete this stage of their education. Also, by so doing, they earn the respect of Harvard physicians who may then sponsor them for medical careers. Interns therefore direct their effort less toward learning than toward providing patient care. Interns, by devoting themselves to doing their job, act in accord with the objectives of the hospital and the purposes of the medical elite.

What I have said so far establishes the context in which I will discuss Harvard internships. Much of what I will say deals with the experiences of young men after they have presented themselves on the wards of the Boston City Hospital. These young men may have only a vague understanding of the phenomenon I call the medical elite. But they do come to be part of the Harvard Medical Unit and, by so doing, are potentially future members of the elite. For that reason, what they must do and how they do it during the internship are an important part of the training of the leaders of American medicine. In addition to questions about the character of an elite segment, other questions I ask are: Why do they come to the Harvard Medical Unit? What kinds of problems do they face as interns, and how do they solve them to their satisfaction and the satisfaction of those with whom they must work?

All internships combine academic and practical activities. Some have more of one kind than the other, depending on the hospitals they are served in. As programs of training, they consist of lectures, conferences, and meetings with practicing physicians. In addition, interns assume responsibility for admitting, examining, prescribing, and caring for the patients assigned to them. Complicating the life of the intern even more is the fact that he must work with members of other occupations at the hospital. These people have their own work to do, and their actions produce working conditions and relationships that facilitate the intern's work. Other workers cannot be expected to arrange their work for his convenience.

The academic and practical experiences of an internship may

conflict. An effort to attend all lectures, conferences, and meetings may leave little time to do what must be done for patients. On the other hand, not all patients contribute to learning. Many patients have the same illness, and attending to them may not provide any new experiences relevant for an internship as interns see it. In circumstances such as I have described, an internship is a "problematic situation," requiring the intern to coordinate his efforts to meet both his need to learn and the demands of the work required of him.

Interns are highly motivated and anticipate doing a great deal of work. Many think they will be able to do it all. But as they try, they learn the facts of working in institutions. The conflicting demands of their situation and the expectations of those with whom they work soon lead them to realize that everything cannot be done and, no matter what is done, not everyone will be satisfied with their efforts. When interns confront this dilemma, they attempt to determine what is an acceptable level of effort and tacitly agree among themselves to take that as their standard for how much to do and on what things to exert effort during the year.

For the purpose of analyzing the level and direction of effort, I use the concepts of interactionist sociology, which assumes that human behavior is reciprocal.[11] People influence those with whom they interact and in turn are influenced by them. In any work situation, people determine a course of action more or less in accord with what others expect and define as appropriate. Although I entered the field with no specific hypotheses, I was committed to the idea that interns would solve the problems they faced by organizing their activity in accordance with the expectations of residents, physicians, nurses, and others with whom they had to work. What I observed were groups of people who interacted with interns, and the ways those groups affected the interns' level and direction of effort by controlling the circumstances in which interns must learn and work.

Some important features of the intern's experiences are specific to his immediate social situation in the training hospital: (1) the

11. The rationale for my study is very much the same as that used by Becker, Geer, Hughes, and Strauss, *Boys in White*.

work others do, particularly when it conflicts with the stated purpose of an internship and requires some sort of unique arrangement between intern and other personnel; (2) the power various work groups have and the way they exercise that power to facilitate their own work and establish working relationships in keeping with the way they think things should be done. These features become major determinants of interns' level and direction of effort.

In my analysis of levels and direction of effort, I am concerned with the circumstances that influence interns as they choose among the many things they could do and decide on particular ways of doing them. People who face many of the same problems frequently have much the same definition of their situation and, in response, collectively evolve a similar course of action. This collective view of a behavior in a particular situation can be called a group perspective.

Perspectives, of course, may be long or short ranged. Long-range perspectives are those that brought the individual into the present situation, for example, the belief that a university-affiliated internship is a prelude to the "right" residency. Faced with specific immediate problems, the intern develops a short-run perspective. Although both kinds will be discussed, I am more concerned with short-run perspectives and deal with long-range goals only as they influence the immediate situation at the training hospital. I will analyze the circumstances in which they arise and the mechanisms by which other hospital work groups play a part in shaping them. These mechanisms—the ideas and actions of others at the hospital—present problems for interns, place restraints on the kind of perspective they can develop, and in other ways influence their thinking and action. The operating perspective that finally emerges results from the interaction between interns and other medical personnel.

The intern depends on others because they have information he needs or can provide services that would facilitate his work. He is not, however, without information of his own, and he has the potential to be a valuable resource. He does, for example, know the patient and can tell other people things they need to know in order to do their own work. These circumstances lend themselves to a model of interaction as social exchange.[12] Using a theory of behavior as exchange, we may assume that the efforts of interns and others to do their work satisfactorily will result in a network of relationships in which the conditions are shaped by the exchange of information, services, and other social goods. [13] The exchanges negotiated will be related to the circumstances of the work setting and the crux of a perspective permitting interns to coordinate their effort at Boston City Hospital.

What I have said in this chapter indicates how I approached the study of the Harvard Medical Unit at the Boston City Hospital. Specifically, I approached the Unit as an elite group of physicians who hold positions from which they control a route to specialty, research, and teaching careers in medicine. My objective is to clarify the processes by which new members of the medical profession are recruited for training, what they must do to satisfactorily complete their training, and the implications of that training for their subsequent medical careers. What follows is a report of my observations and conclusions regarding the social organization of the Unit, and the efforts of young men to make the most of training offered by the medical elite.

12. Stephen J. Miller, "Exchange and Negotiated Learning in Graduate Medical Education," *Sociological Quarterly* (Fall, 1966), pp. 469–479.

13. George C. Homans, "Social Behavior as Exchange," *American Journal of Sociology* (1958), pp. 597–606.

2. Problems and Proof of Observations

WHAT FOLLOWS is a detailed description of what I actually did and how I did it during my time at the Boston City Hospital. It reports the problems I encountered as an observer at the hospital and a statement of the method by which I collected and analyzed my data.

My position at the time I entered the hospital was Assistant Professor of Social Research at Brandeis University. I was not then affiliated with Harvard University, nor was any member of its faculty or staff directly involved in my study. I was simply a member of the Brandeis faculty conducting independent research and teaching sociology.

Although I made some assumptions when I undertook this study, I had no specific hypotheses about how interns would organize their activities, or how other hospital personnel might influence their efforts. The assumption that the actions of interns would be a product of their interaction with others at the hospital did not allow me to state specific hypotheses before

I knew something about the relationships among those people. Assuming, as I did, that the character of the Harvard Medical Unit would be emergent, a result of the interaction among people, it would have been illogical to proceed as though the internship were a constant set of relationships dictated by the prescriptions of medical education. My research problem, as I originally saw it, was to discover the patterned relationships by observing what actually did happen to young men during a year at Boston City Hospital.

The problem led me to adopt the method of participant observation. I put on a white coat and took part in the interns' daily life. I went where they went and, whenever possible, did what they did. The study extended over eighteen months. During that time I openly observed what happened, listened to what was said, and questioned people at the hospital. As I gathered data, it became obvious that the internship could not be divorced from other activity at the Harvard Medical Unit or from the Unit's particular place in American medicine.

The most important source of data was direct observation of interns' and others' behavior on the wards, at clinics, and during conferences, lectures, and meetings. I spent a great deal of time walking around and talking casually with interns as they worked. After introducing myself to the staff, I was able to walk freely into the ward and join a group of interns. I frequently selected a single intern and spent a day with him. If, for example, he left the ward to attend a conference, I went with him. While he was on the ward, I watched whatever he was doing. I could thus observe activity directly and ask on-the-spot questions about what interns did and why they did it.

I had no problem gaining entry to the Harvard Medical Unit; my study had the physicians' approval. Two Harvard physicians who participated in the initial planning continued to serve as consultants throughout my stay at Boston City Hospital. Needless to say, I could not have conducted the study without their support of my work. I am grateful that the physicians with whom I collaborated understood that they could best assist me by allowing me to make my own way at the hospital, while affording me the benefits of their knowledge and years of experience in medicine. Other physicians, trying to be helpful, suggested specific topics they thought would interest me, but at no time did any physician place any restriction on where I could go or attempt to limit my inquiry in any way. Once satisfied that I had a legitimate purpose, they did not interfere. I was free to observe and talk to anyone who might give me information or otherwise assist my study.

Although I had no trouble getting in, I did have a problem establishing myself as an independent observer. People could not at first accept me without fear that I was a spy or gathering information for a report similar to Abraham Flexner's.[1] I also had some trouble fitting into the hospital routine. At the beginning, when I did join an intern for the day, he would often stop what he was doing so we could talk. Since I wanted to observe the content of his daily work, his attempts to cooperate with me defeated my purpose. I therefore had to find ways to fit myself into his routine without interrupting him. Despite my efforts, at the outset of my field work I was in the way because there was nothing for me to do.

I made no attempt to keep my study a secret, and interns knew I was there to observe and question them about their experiences. It was therefore important to know how people saw me and whether they believed that certain kinds of information and events should be kept from me. In that regard, my first days in the field were uncomfortable. When I approached, conversations would stop, or groups would disperse, or interns would try to lose me in the corridors. More than one intern asked me to wait for him and never returned. Experiences of this sort are often reported by participant-observers attempting to establish themselves in an organization or community. I was an intruder, and people felt ill at ease with me until they determined to their own satisfaction who I was.

My problems in the field were greater than could normally be expected. When I began my work, I did not know about an

1. Abraham Flexner conducted a study of medical education in the United States and Canada. His method was to go to the medical school and talk with physicians and their students. Abraham Flexner, *Medical Education in the United States and Canada, Bull.* #4 (New York, Carnegie Foundation for the Advancement of Teaching, 1910).

existing conflict between house officers and the hospital administration. That conflict, I later learned, was one of the factors contributing to my initial difficulty. In 1964 the administrators were having difficulty with an organization of interns and residents at the hospital. Many had complained about antiquated facilities, insufficient nursing personnel, and inadequate salaries. The House Officer's Association had recently negotiated a salary raise and had retained lawyers to negotiate for further increases, additional parking, and improvement of working conditions. A committee representing interns and residents had raised these issues with the administration. At the time, several official accrediting bodies were reviewing the hospital's facilities and the type and quality of its services. Although the focus of these investigations was not the quality of the training offered, the Internship Review Committee of the Council of Medical Education, which was concerned with the quality of training, would take their findings into consideration when approving training programs at the hospital. In other words, much of what was happening could jeopardize the program's approved status. The House Officer's Association was actively attempting to inform the public about working conditions at the hospital, but many interns and residents were understandably fearful of finding themselves at a hospital that was not approved. I thus entered the hospital at a less than opportune time to begin my study.

My field work was made still more difficult by some unwanted publicity. Local newspapers reported that I had been "selected as personal observer," to "record all aspects of the internship, ranging from the intern's attitude toward his superiors, fellows, and library facilities, to his level of medical knowledge, diagnostic ability, therapeutic skill, and management competence." [2] This and the publication of a similar item in a newsletter published by the hospital for employees and staff served to identify me with the hospital administration.[3]

2. "Harvard, Brandeis Eye Intern," Boston *Sunday Herald,* July 5, 1964.

3. See *The BCH Progress Notes,* Special Centennial Issue, Summer, 1964.

Although Harvard physicians had explained to interns and residents who I was, many people distrusted me. I think that in the beginning they concealed a great deal from me. I would like to say that I overcame my problems by astute field methods and intelligent explanation of myself and the study. In fact, many of my problems resolved themselves because of circumstances over which I had no control.

When the study was originally planned, it was with the co-operation and approval of Harvard, whose physicians gave me permission to do my work and informed the hospital's administrators of the study. In the interim, however, the hospital administration had changed, and when I arrived some administrators did not know about me or the purpose of my study. When some of these men finally did learn I was in the hospital, I had to present myself to them and obtain their permission to continue the work. Before that happened, however, interns and residents became aware that administration did not know who I was.

Shortly after the newspaper stories appeared, interns had been requested to meet with one of the hospital's administrators. Not knowing the purpose of this meeting, they tried to find out by questioning a senior resident. During the discussion an intern complained about the work of aides on the wards. "How," he asked, "do you go about replacing those people?" The senior resident laughed and said, "You don't!" He went on to explain that when he was an assistant resident, he wanted an aide fired and was almost fired himself. The intern looked perturbed and asked, "You mean you were a house officer and almost got fired because of an aide?" The senior resident nodded, adding as an afterthought: "You have to watch who you take on." Another intern told the group a head nurse had told him that one of the aides had tenure, but she did not. We all laughed, but one of the interns said he thought I had more tenure than a senior resident. At that point, we were joined by a secretary, who told the resident that everyone had been notified of the meeting. An intern, looking at me, said, "I think he is the only one that knows what the meeting is about." Interns obviously suspected me.

Later that day I joined the interns at the administrator's office. The administrator was not in his office, and the intern I had walked over with said, to no one in particular, "Well, the least we can do is sit down and wait for the man, but I'm sure he hasn't anything important to say." While we waited, my companion asked me a number of questions about hospital administration and administrators. Since I knew little about either, I shrugged my shoulders. A few minutes later the administrator entered and, after looking at my name tag, greeted me as "Dr. Miller." He identified every person in the room in the same way. We followed him into his office, which was air-conditioned. An intern who had earlier complained about hot conference rooms asked why he did not "do this for the entire hospital." Looking around his office, our host informed us that there were plans to refurbish the entire hospital; he explained that his office had been decorated before he came. Turning to the intern who had asked the question, I asked him if it wasn't the air-conditioning, he was referring to, not the paneling, furniture, and fresh paint. "Yes," he replied, "I was, but see how guilty he is?"

We listened as the administrator discussed a number of items on his agenda. What was said is less important than the fact that many of the man's comments were directed at me. For example, he mentioned the rumors that house officers were taking food from the trays on the wards. Possibly he assumed me to be the most likely culprit because of my size: I am well over six feet tall and outweighed every other person in the room by at least fifty pounds. Looking at me, he said he was certain none of us was involved, but cautioned us against eating on the wards. In fact, none of us had been doing so, but after that I never refused a cup of coffee or a piece of cake when a nurse or an intern offered it. It became clear as the meeting progressed that the administrator did not know who I was. That fact amused the interns and worked very much in my favor. A number of them leaned toward me during the meeting and asked if I was doing anything about the Blood Bank's need for blood; if I was worried about malpractice charges; and if I planned to bring any problems I had with patients to the attention of this administrator. After the meeting the interns moaned and gave vent to outspoken criticism of administrators in general and this one in particular. One said, "I've got nothing better to do than come over here and let this jerk shit on me." Another turned to me and said, "You should do a study of hospital administrators."

For a time my presence at the hospital continued as a source of amusement to interns since others besides administrators did not know who I was. When dressed in the white coat worn by interns and residents, there was no obvious way to distinguish me from other Harvard personnel at the hospital. More than once a nurse ran up to me, asking what she should do for a critical patient, and all I could do was point to an intern or resident or suggest she get a doctor. At other times teaching physicians who thought they remembered me from the fourth year at Harvard Medical School asked me questions. When I was unable to answer, and before I had a chance to explain, they covered my embarrassment and questioned someone else. At least one physician apologized for so embarrassing me, saying he was sure that I knew the answer because I had done so well as a clinical clerk at another Harvard-affiliated hospital. I am certain that there are people who, if asked, would name me as the laziest and least intelligent young man ever to serve an internship at the Boston City Hospital.

Finally the interns joined in the fun at my expense. To this day I do not know which one pointed me out to visiting physicians as a "big man in medicine," thus forcing me into a lengthy explanation of who I was to someone anxious to talk to one of the "big names." That kind of incident occurred most frequently during and shortly after the hospital centennial, when many alumni returned to visit. At least one other intern delighted in telling the story of the administrator who roamed the wards at night looking for a "fat intern stealing food from patients." All of these incidents, of course, helped to establish me as an independent observer, certainly as nothing more threatening than a sociologist.

When administrators did become aware of my presence, they asked me to meet with them and discuss the study. Thus I came face to face with administrators who had seen me around the hospital and thought me to be an intern. Much to their credit, they took this in almost good humor and allowed me to continue my work.

Almost no one could suspect that I was a stooge for the administration after it became apparent that they had no more knowledge of my presence and purpose than many others did. Another problem, however, was some residents' fear that I was gathering information for another Flexner report, or at least a report that would be critical of medical education at the hospital. A senior resident suggested that it might be wise for me to meet with a few of the assistant residents and explain my work. If I was to continue at the hospital, it was necessary that these men who have charge of the wards also accept me. If they didn't, there was much they could keep hidden or could instruct interns to conceal from me. Needless to say, I took the first opportunity to arrange a meeting with the assistant residents on the wards I was studying.

The following excerpt from my field notes describes how my meeting with assistant residents was arranged, illustrating their concerns about the study.

> Yanofsky and I were on our way back to the ward from lunch. He asked me how the study was going. Yanofsky and Bloom [assistant residents] had asked about the study repeatedly during the past week. I said that I heard Bloom was also interested in the study. He nodded, I suggested that we get together and talk, if they had the time. Yanofsky said he would very much like to do so but had hesitated to ask me for a meeting. We arranged a time to meet. When we entered the ward a nurse stopped me and asked: "By the way, how do you like studying interns?" Yanofsky was still with me. I said I was having fun and enjoyed my work. She asked: "Do you put in your notes that they drink coffee all the time?" I said that they didn't and she laughed, saying, "I know, I was just teasing you."

My relationships with interns and nurses were relaxed by that time, and I was occasionally being put on about my encounters with administrators and physicians who thought me to be an intern. There was very little such joking with assistant residents. It was almost another week before I made note of any such humor between myself and an assistant resident.

> I was sitting in the laboratory, talking with the interns. Yanofsky entered and sat down at a desk. He picked up a newspaper and nodded to me. After reading for a moment or so, he turned to me and said: "How about that? They're going to transfer your study!" I think I jumped, because I have been thinking of going over to the other wards but did not want to do so before handling some of the problems that the recent newspaper articles had caused between me and the assistant residents. I asked what he meant and he laughed, saying, "I mean Vietnam, of course. We may all be draftees and that means you will have to go with us." I laughed, but it reminded me that Yanofsky, though always courteous, has given me the feeling that I am intruding on whatever he or others are doing. This was the first time he attempted to be funny, even by making a remark that may well be hostile.

That same day, I met with assistant residents to talk about the study.

At this meeting the assistant residents asked two questions. What kinds of data are you collecting? Will you publish your study? I told them that the study would be published because many people were interested in the subject, and publications helped my career. Yanofsky did not hear what I had said and asked Bloom. Laughing, Bloom said: "He said it won't help his career if he doesn't publish the study." Yanofsky looked at me and said: "At least you're honest about it." My response to the question had been almost word for word what I had heard many Harvard physicians say about their own research. Asked to elaborate further on my work, "without compromising the study," I responded: "We would like to know what interns learn, who they learn it from, and what they do with what they learn."

Yanofsky cautioned me that what they did learn was more than "book learning." He gave examples of what I will in subsequent chapters refer to as "learning the ropes." Yanofsky then asked if I was aware that many people resented the study. In his words:

> People don't like it. I know that I resent it when you come around. I am pretty busy and have a lot of work to do. I don't like someone hanging around. People don't like it. After a while it doesn't bother you, but it does for a while. Find something to do with yourself, that should help.

The meeting ended in this way:

> Yanofsky asked, "When do you think you'll publish the study?" I told him that I had at least two years of data collection, but that I would see he received a copy no matter where he was at the time. I said jokingly, "Well, I don't want to keep you from whatever you have to do. If you have any other questions, I'll be happy to answer them." Yanofsky smiled and said, "Well, things aren't too bad."

Though I had made every effort not to be, apparently I was in the way because there was nothing for me to do. When I returned to the wards, therefore, I looked for ways to help interns with their work. If, for example, a patient had to be weighed, I would go for the scale. There were many such things that I could get, carry, and push, thus saving the interns an extra trip or some time. Also, I could help out by positioning the patient during a procedure or physical examination. These chores became a continuing part of my activity as an observer. This is not to say that I did very much but that I did whatever I was asked to do to help an intern with his work. Many times there was nothing for me to do. The field notes, however, contain numerous descriptions of my talking with waiting patients, pushing scales, carrying charts, finding nurses, helping move or lift a patient, and in other ways making myself useful. Also, interns have to make many trips off the wards. They have to run from place to place arranging for services and finding people who can help them with their work. When others were busy, I was always available to accompany them. As I came to be accepted and tried to make myself useful, most interns were happy to have me around. The following comments, for example, were made by an intern who earlier in the year had tried to lose me every time I attempted to observe him at work:

I went to the house officers' dining room, where I met Rosengard and Butler. I put together a tray and joined them at a table. As I sat down, Rosengard asked, "Where are you?" I told him I was spending most of my time at the clinic but would come over and visit him if he really missed me. Rosengard, shaking his head, "No, thanks. Stay where you are. I'm very happy on the ward."

He turned to Butler and asked if I had ever watched him at work. Butler said, "No, not really. Why?" Rosengard: "You haven't been watched until you've been watched by him. It's weird! He not only watches you, but if you take off, he meets you at places. I'm glad he's watching other people now." Butler asked him if I was really that bad. He laughed and said, "No, almost but not really. At least he's good company . . ."

I asked Rosengard if he was happy being back on wards. He replied, "It's good to be back, after the clinic." I shrugged and asked, "Is that all you have to say?" Rosengard: "What do you want? You didn't buy lunch!" He laughed and, walking away, turned to say, "I'm on Peabody 2. Come up and see me some time."

In summary, at the outset people had their own explanations of my presence and of the study. What they told me or allowed me to see almost certainly depended on their opinions of me and my purpose there. Although events in time established me as an independent observer, curiosity about me complicated my relationships with others. They may, of course, have only needed time to get used to me. But many events and circumstances did lend credence to the early notion that I was a spy. For that reason I decided to repeat my first few months' observations during the following year. To learn the hospital's routine and acquaint myself with its ecology, I had entered the field a month before the group I was to study arrived. I used observations made during that time to develop initial hypotheses about the problems of an internship. Whatever questions the events I have described raised about the validity of those observations are, in my opinion, answered by the fact that I repeated them later. By the end of my first summer at the hospital, interns and assistant residents had accepted me. My observations now afforded me an opportunity to document the assistant residents' experience and to follow up those data by questioning them about what was happening.

My original plan was to follow the groups of interns on two medical services through an entire sequence of experiences on the wards and at the outpatient clinics. This plan, I believed, would permit observation of all situations during the year. I soon learned, however, that interns did not remain in fixed groups. They were assigned as individuals, and new groups were formed almost monthly. In other words, there was no one group of interns, but many small groups whose activities differed at different times of the year. Staying on the wards would have permitted me to observe all interns, as each of them spent a certain amount of time there. But while this would have given me extensive coverage of interns, I could not have learned much about their experiences in other situations. Following only a few interns, on the other hand, would permit observation of all situations, but not of all interns. This would have prevented my noting individual differences that might account for the character of their relationships and the level and direction of their effort.

I finally decided to spend time with as many groups as possible, but not to follow any particular interns from the wards to the clinic. I would, for example, spend time on the female ward of the Second Medical Service and then later move on to the outpatient clinic. Some of the interns I had previously observed might be reassigned, but though I might observe them again, the situation would be different. My plan, then, allowed me to cover all situations—that is, the wards, clinics, accident and admitting floors—and to observe a more or less random sample of interns. Situational observations afforded opportunities to document the experiences of most interns, even though I observed some more often than others. This, I thought, was more valuable than seeing the year as only a few interns saw it.

I moved from group to group, went to lectures and conferences, and spent time on the admitting ward and at the clinic much as the interns did. I accompanied them on rounds with visiting physicians, sat in on their discussions, and watched individual interns with patients. Thus, I participated in all their activities without necessarily seeing each one in all situations.

In the beginning, I put everything I saw in my notes and recorded in detail all conversations I took part in or overheard. After I had described things to my satisfaction, I began to leave out what I already knew or had observed many times. For example, I described the physical facilities of the place only once and, after a time, recorded the routine of a physical examination only if it differed in some way from others I had seen. When I had data, I formulated an explanation of the way I thought some things happened. Then I gathered additional data, which supported or disproved those explanations. I thought, for example, that medical students who had been at the hospital before the interns came were affecting the level and direction of interns' efforts by using their knowledge to influence what inexperienced newcomers did and how they did it. When I had sufficient data to substantiate the explanation of the student-intern relationship, I no longer recorded all supporting incidents. I continued, however, to record any negative cases.

My field notes consist of data that were important because of my particular interest at the time and other data unrelated to my interests but a part of what was happening. I was not, for example, interested in the work of X-ray technicians, but I did record all that I saw of their work. Later observations suggested a relationship between interns and X-ray technicians similar to that between students and interns earlier in the year. By searching my notes for what I had already recorded about the technicians, I was able to substantiate an explanation that had been formulated after my field work at the hospital.

Although I was studying a university-affiliated internship, I was interested in internships in general. For that reason I arranged to study interns at a Boston community general hospital conducting an approved program of graduate medical education. My method there was also participant observation. This second set of observations allowed me to gather comparative data as well as to question other people about explanations I had evolved at the Boston City Hospital. I wanted to know, for example, if medical students were really as important to interns as I had come to believe. Since the community hospital had no medical students, I could discover how their absence made the internship different. What I found indicated that the absence of medical students made some difference in how quickly interns learned their jobs. Although nurses at the community hospital served the function of students at Boston City, nurses did not know the work of an intern so well as students did and were, therefore, less able to assist inexperienced interns.

In general, I used the community hospital as a place to determine what was common about the internships I was studying. My observations at that hospital also served to point out processes that may be unique to the university-affiliated hospital conducting research as well as training physicians and providing patient services. I describe in Chapter 3 the research facilities at Boston City Hospital, but it was the lack of such facilities at the community general hospital that first made me aware that the organization of a hospital for research purposes was in part the result of a phenomenon that could not be divorced from the experiences of interns. That phenomenon is the existence of the medical elite as I have described it. At the community hospital there was no evidence that an internship was anything more than a straightforward year of hospital training before a young man became a practicing physician or chose a specialty in which to continue his training. On the other hand, internship at Boston City Hospital was apparently an integral part of the organization of the medical elite and drew meaning from its place in that organization.

After observing and questioning interns at both hospitals, I formulated questions relevant to the students' decisions to intern at a university-affiliated rather than a general hospital. A preliminary analysis of earlier data led me to hypothesize that students who chose Harvard internships had been sponsored by alumni of the Harvard Medical Unit. Knowing that working conditions at Boston City Hospital would not be the best, they chose those internships for reasons related to their career aspirations and were influenced in their choice by physicians who knew the implications of a Harvard internship for a medical career.

My data indicated that interns at the community general

hospital had based their choice on such criteria as hospital facilities, working conditions, pay, and the kinds of patients they would be attending. Harvard interns apparently tended to overlook these things. If this was so, I wanted to know why, and what other criteria influenced interns to come to Boston City Hospital before they became directly acquainted with the Harvard Medical Unit. After a few weeks at the hospital interns all know of its reputation for teaching and research. My interest was whether or not they knew of this before applying and whether such knowledge affected their choice of an internship in any way. For this purpose, I formulated a questionnaire and sent it to medical students who chose Boston City Hospital.

In addition to the methods described, I also gathered data through many formal interviews of interns, assistant residents, and nurses. During my field work I arranged such interviews whenever I needed elaboration of information acquired by observation. Thus I was also able to obtain information from people I did not often see in the wards or at the clinics. I did not see the chief resident, for example, and had to arrange interviews to obtain whatever information I wanted from him. Another such informant was the visiting physician who came to the clinics to work with students; I had few occasions to talk with him. With people such as these I had to arrange interviews by appointment. Others, such as nurses, whom I saw day in and day out, I could interview casually on the spot, as I needed answers to my questions. Some people I did not expect to interview approached me and themselves arranged for me to talk with them. Many of these conversations—with elevator operators, charwomen, and other personnel—resulted in useful information about the hospital, its history, and the medical schools conducting training programs there. Near the end of the year I conducted formal interviews with almost all the interns. This served two purposes: (1) to determine the educational backgrounds of the interns I observed and to elicit information relative to their choice of an internship and their future plans; and (2) to question interns I had not often observed about their experiences and to check my observations against what they told me. Based on the results of data already collected and analyzed, I designed these interviews either to verify my own explanations or particular points or to check them against how respondents said things worked. In each interview I asked for examples, sometimes presenting my own definitions of situations and discussing with the interns how these differed from their own interpretations.[4] If there were discrepancies or refutations of my explanations, I made it a point to gather additional data during the remainder of the year.

As I gathered data, I attempted to organize it topically, according to my interests. After a few months, however, the data were pertinent to different topics. The records of my field notes and interviews consist of approximately 2,000 single-spaced typed pages. Although the material could have been subdivided by topics or organized in terms of the groups observed, these methods did not lend themselves to an analysis of the entire year. I kept notes and interviews in chronological order. An indexing system allowed me to locate any given topic, group, or situation as needed for a qualitative analysis of the data.

I did part of the analysis during my stay at the hospital. That is, I evolved numerous tentative explanations of what was happening on the basis of incomplete field data. Most of the analysis, however, was done after I had completed my field work. My effort in the field was devoted to discovering interns' problems and documenting their solutions. After leaving the hospital, I organized my explanations into a series of hypotheses. A hypothesis, for my purposes, was a best guess of the way something operated at the hopital.

My major analytical problem was to assess the evidence I had to support the hypotheses I evolved from the data I had collected. In assessing hypotheses with qualitative data, I tried to determine the probability that a hypothesis correctly stated the circumstances and conditions found at Boston City Hospital. What I did was to gather all the evidence in support of a partic-

4. The rationale for my interviewing techniques may be found in Arnold M. Rose, "A Research Note on Interviewing," *American Journal of Sociology,* LI (September, 1945), pp. 143–144; and Howard S. Becker, "Field Methods and Techniques, A Note on Interviewing Tactics," *Human Organization,* 12, 4 (Winter, 1954), pp. 31–32.

ular hypothesis and compare that to the evidence that could refute it or require me to change it to take into account any negative cases that appeared in my field notes.[5]

The data were recorded observations, made by myself. If the observations were to stand as evidence for my hypotheses, the data had to be collated, catalogued, and related to the hypotheses.[6] The purpose of data analysis, therefore, was to relate the hypotheses evolved to data collected in the field. All the data in support of a hypothesis were collated and all other data were searched for negative cases. That is, I made an effort to refute the hypothesis by collating all exceptions to the rule implied by the hypothesis. I considered any exception that could not be explained to be sufficient reason for rejecting the hypothesis or changing it so that no unexplained exceptions remained in the data. If the evidence in support of a particular hypothesis was not contradicted by other data, the hypothesis was accepted. For any particular hypothesis, then, there were recorded observations that supported its acceptance.

Though a hypothesis had been accepted, I further compared it to all other hypotheses of its set; a set consisted of all hypotheses evolved in explanation of a particular phenomenon. When a significant set of hypotheses had been established, I compared to the set itself other sets of accepted hypotheses. My purpose in doing so was to determine the consistency of explanations by searching for contradictions within and between sets of accepted hypotheses. I could in this way relate hypotheses to each other in much the same way that hypotheses had been related to data collected in the field. This is not so much a test of hypotheses as it is a test of the hypothetical model which could be generalized from explanatory hypotheses. If the hypotheses within a

5. This method of analysis is discussed in William Foote Whyte, "Observational Field Work Methods," in Jahoda, Deutsch, and Cook, eds., *Research Methods in Social Relations*, II (New York, Dryden Press, 1951), pp. 493–514; and Howard S. Becker, Blanche Geer, Everett C. Hughes, and Anselm Strauss, *Boys in White* (Chicago, University of Chicago Press, 1961), pp. 22, 30–32.

6. A discussion on the procedure for relating hypotheses to data appears in William N. Stephens, *Hypotheses and Evidence* (New York, Thomas Y. Crowell Co., 1968). See particularly, "A System for Judging Evidence," pp. 21–76.

set and between sets of hypotheses do not contradict each other, then they may be asserted together as an explanation of the observed phenomenon.

What I report in subsequent chapters are generalizations based on numerous hypotheses I have accepted about what I observed at Boston City Hospital. None of the hypotheses by themselves afforded a complete explanation of a Harvard internship, but when reported together they clarify the processes by which young men are recruited and prepared for academic rather than practice careers, and document the character of the phenomena I refer to as the elite of the medical profession.

3. The Harvard Unit at Boston City Hospital

THE MODERN physician holds a variety of hospital posts and, when possible, usually associates himself with a medical school. He may be a medical scientist, teacher, or practitioner, but no matter what medical career a modern physician chooses, he will conduct his business within the medical institutions of a community.[1]

The most familiar medical institution is the general hospital established for the delivery of medical care and providing paramedical facilities for the specialized treatment of patients by physicians. Internships and residencies are the means by which many of these hospitals recruit the graduates of approved medical schools to attend patients and provide medical care, thereby assisting practicing physicians.[2]

1. Oswald Hall, "The Stages of a Medical Career," *American Journal of Sociology,* 53, 5 (March, 1948), pp. 327–336.
2. Basil S. Georgopoulos and Floyd C. Mann, *The Community General Hospital* (New York, Macmillan, 1962), p. 5.

The university hospitals affiliated with a medical school share to a greater degree the threefold objective of medical schools: (1) teaching medical students and training physicians; (2) conducting basic research and clinical experimentation; and (3) the delivery of medical care to a population of patients with a diversity of illnesses and complicated medical problems. Like general hospitals, university hospitals recruit medical school graduates to attend patients and provide medical care while learning and gaining experience. Moreover, internships and residencies afford medical schools an opportunity to select and sponsor young men for careers in medicine.

Most medicine in Boston is in some way affiliated with one of three medical schools: Boston University, Tufts University, and Harvard Medical School. Each has teaching, research, and service agreements with hospitals and other medical settings throughout the city. Although institutions remain autonomous, hospitals affiliated with a medical school are closely linked by reciprocal agreements, working relationships, and the colleague-ship of physicians in the various medical settings. The physicians on the staff of a given hospital are likely to hold faculty appointments at a particular medical school.

Excluding unaffiliated hospitals and those united by the religious orders, Boston medicine is conducted in three sets of medical settings, each affiliated with a medical school.[3] All hospitals, clinics, and laboratories affiliated with a medical school comprise a subsystem of local medicine. The institutions of a particular subsystem subscribe to a single body of policies governing the practice of medicine and the delivery of medical care, and their staff physicians have compatible opinions about medicine and the medical profession. The teaching and practice of medicine are distributed among these subsystems of institutions and subgroups of physicians, each of which differs to some degree from the others in policy and opinion, so that each has a unique subculture of its own.

3. The "more important" hospitals are affilated with one of the three Boston medical schools. Others, until now unaffiliated, seek or have negotiated affiliations; for example, the Cambridge City Hospital has recently become affiliated with the Harvard Medical School. Also, community hospitals in the Boston suburbs have made overtures to the medical schools.

The Department of Medicine of the Harvard Medical School is an association of physician groups at four Boston hospitals: Massachusetts General Hospital, Peter Bent Brigham Hospital, Beth Israel Hospital, and Boston City Hospital. I observed only the interns on the Second and Fourth Medical Services, where patient care is provided under Harvard auspices and which, with the research divisions of the Thorndike Memorial Laboratory, make up the Harvard Medical Unit at Boston City Hospital.

BOSTON CITY HOSPITAL

Boston City Hospital, according to its brochure, is "one of the great general hospitals of the world, opened to the people of Boston on June 1, 1864." During that first year the hospital had a visiting staff of six surgeons and six physicians and a house staff of five interns, who had been selected from the undergraduates of Harvard Medical School. "The first group of interns were not drawn from the graduating class of Harvard," newcomers to the hospital are told, "but from the undergraduates because the graduating class was going to war—the Civil War, that is." [4] Later in 1864, Harvard began teaching medical students at Boston City Hospital.

"Originally in 1864," wrote William B. Castle, a distinguished Harvard Professor of Medicine, "twenty-eight beds for medical patients were provided on each of three wards, E, F, and G, located in [one] of two pavilions . . . E and G were used for male, F for female patients, and the basement beneath served as a medical outpatient department." [5] Today the hospital is a

4. Welcoming remarks to interns on the Second and Fourth (Harvard) Medical Services, June 26, 1964. The Alumni Day audience, May 29, had been told: "As the graduating class of the Harvard Medical School had largely entered the Union Army and Navy Services, the hospital staff chose five undergraduate students as house officers."

5. William B. Castle, M.D., was the first Francis Weld Peabody Faculty Professor and had been the George Richards Minot Professor of Medicine at the Harvard Medical School as well as Director of the Thorndike Medical Laboratory and the Second and Fourth (Harvard) Medical Services at Boston City Hospital. I rely on his history of the Harvard Medical Unit at the Hospital, "The Second and Fourth (Harvard) Medical Services and the Thorndike Memorial Laboratory," in John J. Byrne, ed., *A History of the Boston City Hospital: 1905–1964* (Boston, Sheldon Press, 1964), pp. 57–90.

facility of a thousand or more beds for research, teaching, and care of Boston's medically indigent. In 1864 it boasted a total medical staff of 17; today it has more than 400 physicians and surgeons and 300 interns, residents, and research fellows.[6]

The hospital is a complex of buildings connected by tunnels and corridors leading to myriad offices, laboratories, and wards. Although attempts have been made to modernize the buildings, gossip hints that the city is making every effort to maintain the hospital as a historic site in its original condition. In 1964, the year of the Boston City Hospital Centennial, an intern informed a less knowing visitor whom he met in an elevator that Sherman had started his March to the Sea at the time the hospital's doors were opened. The elevator operator interjected, "What d'ya mean at the same time? He started his march at the City [Boston City Hospital]!" The hospital does, in fact, look as if it had been allowed to deteriorate. The physical facilities are often make-do; the buildings are old and in need of repair. This is not to say that the facilities are not adequate. Rather, at least, they are not modern.

Harvard, Boston University, and Tufts operate training and research units at Boston City. Each school staffs medical services, as well as the outpatient clinics. The Harvard Medical School maintains the Second and Fourth Medical Services consisting of two male and two female wards, the Fifth Surgical Service, and the special services of psychiatry, neurology, and neurosurgery, as well as the Thorndike Memorial Laboratory where Harvard physicians conduct a variety of medical research. In addition, each of the three medical schools supports programs of teaching and research of particular interest to its physicians. All such programs are more or less associated with one of the specialty outpatient clinics: cardiology, dermatology, diabetes,

6. When Dr. Wiliam Castle became Associate Director of the Thorndike Memorial Laboratory in 1932, research fellows were known as residents. Subsequently, the title was changed to connote the difference in place and type of work; that is, research fellows are assigned to work for a year or more in clinical research at the Thorndike Laboratoy; residents are assigned to the staff of the medical services for further clinical training and assume responsibility for the administration of the wards.

endocrinology, or gastroenterology. The Harvard program in diabetes and metabolism, for example, collaborates with the hospital's Diabetes Clinic.

With the exception of the surgical services, each unit is responsible for a variety of medical activities. First, it must staff and supervise the medical care of the acutely ill on its male and female wards. The medical services treat approximately 3,000 patients admitted to these wards during the year. They also operate open clinics for outpatients and follow-up clinics for the continuing care of discharged patients. In rotation the three medical services supply interns and residents who examine and give emergency treatment to patients on the accident floor and in the admitting department. Finally, the physicians of each medical school provide consultation in their specialties to other physicians at the hospital. For example, the Infectious Disease Research Division of the Harvard Medical School and the Fifth and Sixth Medical Services of the Boston University School of Medicine conduct regularly scheduled consultation rounds on infectious diseases. In turn, the Second and Fourth (Harvard) Medical Services have X-ray conferences with a professor of radiology from Boston University.

During 1960 Boston City Hospital's 1,392 beds were occupied by 32,053 patients treated by 700 physicians from three medical schools; another 274,339 patients visited the outpatient department, and 125,000 were treated as emergency cases in the accident and admitting departments.

Many of the patients come from Boston's South End. Before the family of the fictional late George Apley (1866–1933) moved to fashionable Beacon Street, they lived for a few years in the South End. At the time, "nearly everyone was under the impression that this district would be one of the most solid residential sections of Boston instead of becoming, as it is today, a region of rooming houses and worse." [7] But by 1936, when Marquand's memoir of a Boston gentleman was published, the South End had already declined. Today it comprises rooming

7. John P. Marquand, *The Late George Apley* (Boston, Little, Brown, 1936), p. 25.

houses and apartment buildings with absentee landlords, mixed in with industry, bars, cafes, and skid row.[8]

Many people with jobs live and own homes in the South End. Some of its middle class residents cherish visions of "making over the South End into a Georgetown of sorts."[9] But many more are poor, and some live in public housing. Twenty-five per cent of the South End's people are sixty years old or older; they live in cheap rooming houses or crowded apartments. The state has issued 116 liquor licenses in the South End, and the local War on Poverty includes a treatment and rehabilitation center for alcoholics operated by Boston University.[10] The neighborhood's old and poor, as well as its skid row population, receive most of their medical attention at "The City."

The City is, by the nature of its patient population, a medical facility for the acutely ill alcoholic, a geriatric facility for the chronically ill, and a social welfare agency. The alcoholic, according to an intern on the Second Medical Service, "comes to the Accident Floor by police ambulance, or is dragged in by friends, or just comes walking in acutely ill." Patients who are sixty years old or older also come in off the street or are brought from rooming houses by the police. Others come every Friday afternoon, sent by nursing homes in the belief that some medical problem will erupt over the weekend. These patients may stay in the hospital for weeks before returning to the original nursing home or getting located at another one. As one intern said:

> Well, let's put it this way: There are certain patients, those who are chronically ill, that stay with you for a very long time.

8. The skid row of Boston in the South End is an area bounded by Northampton Street on the south, Broadway on the north, Tremont on the west, and Harrison Avenue on the east. A discussion of Boston's skid row is presented by Harold W. Demone and Edward Blacker, "The Unattached and Socially Isolated Residents of Skid Row," Action for Boston Community Development, 1961.

9. "The South End Today," *Boston Magazine* (October, 1965), published by the Greater Boston Chamber of Commerce.

10. The Boston Redevelopment Authority provided statistics and other information about the South End Urban Renewal Area. In 1966, I was contemplating a study of the careers of welfare recipients and held many preliminary interviews with people living in the South End. Boston City Hospital was a major topic of conversation.

If there was a chronic disease hospital associated with the City, where these people could go without having to wait two weeks to have papers processed, it would make life a lot more reasonable . . . The fact of the matter is that they are going to be in the hospital for three weeks anyway, until they get placed [in a nursing home.][11]

Most of these patients are seriously ill and require a great deal of care. For the intern this situation is fortunate, because it affords him exceptional opportunities for studying diseases and obtaining clinical experience. During my first day in the field, for example, I observed a young woman with typhoid.[12] I was told that an intern might see a case or two, "but not really many more than that, maybe not even that many [and] he might not see any." [13] Patients of this sort are the unique and, for that reason, the "interesting" ones, and word of them is passed around the hospital. The great majority of patients, however, have more common chronic and acute illness.

THE HARVARD MEDICAL UNIT

In 1915 Boston City Hospital's trustees decided that the administrative heads of the Third and Fourth Medical Services would be appointed on the advice of Tufts and Harvard universities. Thus the new Fourth Medical Service became Harvard affiliated, and its wards, T and U in the Burnham Building, were authorized for Harvard's teaching purposes. Today those wards are Peabody 1 and 2 of the Fourth (Harvard) Medical Service. In 1930 the Second Medical Service became part of the Harvard Medical Unit.

The Second and Fourth Medical Services occupy all of one building and part of another. The Burnham Building, erected in 1906, houses the Fourth; the Medical Building, opened in 1930, houses the Second on the fifth and sixth floors. Each medical

11. Second Medical Service.
12. June 1, 1964. That day, 219 cases of typhoid had been reported in Aberdeen, Scotland.
13. Assistant resident, Medical 5, Second Medical Service, June 1, 1964.

service consists of a male and a female ward with thirty beds each. During a usual year approximately 1,500 patients are admitted to the wards. Their care is entrusted to interns assisted by medical students. The former, in turn, are supervised by residents. The informal hierarchial rule runs this way: A medical service belongs to the senior resident; a ward, to the assistant resident; and the patient, to the intern. On the house staff of the Second and Fourth Medical Services are four senior residents, sixteen assistant residents, and sixteen interns.

Not long after the Fourth Medical Service was opened, Harvard physicians, encouraged by the Dean of the Harvard Medical School, began using the site as an "academic clinic." Massachusetts General and Peter Bent Brigham hospitals had already been established as clinical and research settings. In 1919, supported by a gift in memory of William H. Thorndike, Dr. Francis Weld Peabody became the first director of the Thorndike Laboratory.[14] Under his administration research laboratories were erected, and in November 1923, according to Castle, "the Thorndike Laboratory was formally dedicated and so became the first clinical research facility in a municipal hospital in this country."[15]

Today the laboratory consists of a ward for the study of patients with particular problems, usually transferred from the wards of the medical services, and laboratories occupied by members of the several divisions of research being conducted at the hospital. There are a dozen or more senior investigators, both part- and full-time, and a score of research fellows distributed among nine research divisions.

Although the hospital's patient population may not afford its interns a variety of clinical experiences, it does lend itself to the research divisions. The Division of Liver and Nutrition, for

14. The Harvard Medical Unit has a number of folk heroes. Francis W. Peabody is one, and a lecture of his, "The Care of the Patient," is distributed to all those joining the Harvard Medical Services. Another is Nobel prize-winner George Richards Minot, the "Inquisitive Physician." A folk hero in the making is William B. Castle.

15. William B. Castle, "The Second and Fourth (Harvard) Medical Services and the Thorndike Memorial Laboratory," p. 64.

example, conducts studies of liver disease, particularly cirrhosis, and nutrition in arteriosclerosis conditions that a patient population consisting for the most part of the old and alcoholic amply provides. The many patients admitted with gastrointestinal and other bleeding offer opportunities for studies of the effects of abnormal bleeding, a research concern of the Division of Hemorrhagic Diseases. Other characteristics of the same patient population lend themselves to the various research interests of other divisions of the Thorndike Laboratory.

The work of interns on the Second and Fourth Medical Services consists almost entirely of examining and treating patients admitted to the hospital. Other members of the Unit, however, engage in specialized training or clinical and scientific investigation, and may never examine or treat a patient except for those purposes. Thus there is a wide diversity of positions, duties, and purposes.

Within the hospital, the Harvard physicians foster a subculture with which interns become imbued from the outset. The interns' version of this medical subculture, naturally, differs from that of Harvard physicians, because their duties and purposes are different.[16] But the interns' subculture does reflect the values of Harvard physicians. That is, they agree that training and research are essential purposes of medicine.

The arrangement that the three medical schools have with the City of Boston to occupy Boston City Hospital is not unique. Other schools in other cities share medical settings. Sharing a setting, however, affects the practice of medicine within the hospital. Also, the organization of the hospital that has evolved from the arrangement perpetuates each medical school's subculture of medicine.

Although operating under public auspices, the three private medical schools staff and manage their own medical, surgical, and specialty services. Not only are all hospital departments affiliated with one or more of the schools, but the medical

16. Howard S. Becker, Blanche Geer, Everett C. Hughes, and Anselm L. Strauss, *Boys in White* (Chicago, University of Chicago Press, 1961), pp. 192–193.

schools share the cost of teaching, research, and patient care. During 1964 and 1965 Harvard University, for example, budgeted approximately a million and a half dollars for the cost of maintaining and operating its Unit.[17] Hospital administrators are appointed by the City of Boston. Each medical and surgical service, as well as most departments, however, has an administrative head who is selected from the physicians on the faculty of the particular school with which the service or department is affiliated, or is selected from physicians throughout the country. Thus the director of the Thorndike Laboratory and the Harvard Medical Services is appointed by the trustees of Boston City Hospital, but only on the recommendation of the Dean and faculty of the Harvard Medical School.

The administrative head of a service or department is technically a member of the hospital's administrative staff, but his appointment and the policy that guides him are a result of decisions of physicians responsive to the expectations of colleagues at one of the three medical schools—that is, to their shared understanding of medicine and the medical profession, and of the proper behavior of a physician. Each medical school also selects its own interns, residents, and visiting physicians, who are, only on recommendation of the administrative head of a service or department, appointed by the Board of Trustees to the staff of Boston City Hospital. Thus Harvard, Boston, and Tufts medical schools occupy the hospital and assume much of the responsibility for running their own affairs.

The most obvious consequence of these circumstances is a conflict between the medical schools and the administrators appointed by the city. "Much of the stress and tension occurring in hospitals," writes Croog, "can be traced to varying types of clashes between the [administrative and medical] systems of authority."[18] These clashes result in large part from differences of opinion regarding the problems and purposes of a hospital.

17. Reported by William B. Castle to the Faculty of Medicine, Harvard University, December 18, 1964.

18. Sydney H. Croog, "Interpersonal Relations in Medical Settings," in Howard E. Freeman and others, eds., *Handbook of Medical Sociology* (Englewood Cliffs, Prentice-Hall, 1963), p. 256.

One line of authority is the hospital administration, appointed by the Board of Trustees and responsible for the day-to-day maintenance and operation of the hospital. The other line, the medical staff, is divided among groups of physicians from three medical schools. Because the three schools jointly occupy the hospital, Boston City has more than the two commonly noted lines of authority.[19]

Naturally, additional lines of authority afford more occasions for a clash of interests between the administrative and medical systems. Needless to say, the more occasions for conflict, the more discord. Furthermore, hospital administrators resent the divided loyalties of administrative heads as a subversion of their authority by the medical schools. The shared medical setting heightens the friction between the hospital's administration and its multiple medical staffs.

The hospital comprises three groups of physicians, each with its own understanding of the appropriate concerns of medicine and the activities proper to physicians, and each recruiting or training new physician members. Physicians support divergent opinions on what constitutes the practice of medicine and what its essential purposes are.[20]

The hospital maintains facilities for the training of physicians, scientific investigation, and the treatment of patients, but the three medical schools do not place equal value on these activities. Although the schools attempt to perform each of the tasks creditably, they have somewhat different purposes for being in the hospital. All physicians would agree that the proper concerns of the medical profession are the study and treatment of human diseases. But opinion regarding the relative importance of study and treatment varies greatly, and the opinions of

19. A number of sociologists have delineated the differences between administrative and professional (medical) lines of authority in a hospital. For example, Harvey L. Smith, "Two Lines of Authority: The Hospital's Dilemma," *The Modern Hospital* (March, 1955), pp. 59–64.

20. Physicians are not the only group in agreement with the purpose of hospitals but divided on the essentials of their work. For example, nurses do not agree on what should be the work of a nurse, though they agree that patient care is the purpose of a hospital. See Everett C. Hughes, Helen MacGill Hughes, and Irwin Deutscher, *Twenty-Thousand Nurses Tell Their Story* (Philadelphia, Lippincott, 1958), Chapter 6.

physicians at Boston City Hospital are as varied as those entertained by the medical profession in general.

Each group of physicians at the hospital cherishes a view of medicine not quite like that of the other two. Each group's understanding of medicine unites, in varying combination, the following elements: (1) academic medicine—medicine as the scientific study of human diseases, their nature, causes, and management in the individual patient; (2) traditional medicine —medicine as a private practice with a clientele; and (3) contemporary medicine—medicine as the treatment of patients, as members of a community. One group is only slightly less academic but more contemporary than the Harvard physicians, and the other inclines to a more traditional understanding of medicine. Each of the medical subcultures is a particular version of the general medical culture, emphasizing a somewhat different understanding of the purposes of medicine.

Boston City Hospital fosters a number of conditions necessary for the development of a subculture. For example, each group of physicians is a part of a large group, and its members are congenial by reason of their educational backgrounds, institutional affiliations, and the colleague system. Physicians may be on the hospital staff, but they pride themselves on their faculty appointments at the different medical schools. Also, the physicians of any one group are, by implicit understanding, excluded from participating in the administrative affairs of either of the others. This agreement divides the medical staff and distributes medical responsibilty among three groups rather than entrusting it to a single group. Medical matters, therefore, are not a general concern of a medical staff, but the particular concern of separate groups. Each group may choose its own alternatives and carry on more or less independently. Conditions at the hospital permit each medical school to assume responsibility for its own affairs, particularly teaching and research. They also permit each school to maintain and implement its own understanding of medicine.

A HARVARD SEGMENT OF THE ELITE

My purpose in discussing Boston City Hospital has been to describe the setting in which the Harvard Medical Unit exists: the kind of setting in which interns must work each year. Many medical schools have similar arrangements with hospitals, including the two other medical schools that occupy Boston City Hospital. There is nothing particularly unique about its setting. Also, an academic clinic is not unique in medicine. Groups of physicians staff clinical research facilities at many hospitals affiliated with medical schools. What is different from most other units of this sort is that it is an established segment of the medical profession, whose members have high status and hold institutional positions of power. The Harvard Medical Unit is a distinguishable segment of the medical profession with sufficient prestige and power to be considered a part of the medical elite.

A number of conditions previously postulated must be met for the Harvard Medical Unit to be a segment of the elite. First, its members must share a common understanding of the purposes of medicine. This is not so much a condition for elite status as it is a condition for being a segment. That is, it must be demonstrated that these physicians have similar interests and an agreed upon purpose before they can be considered a segment. Second, the Harvard Medical Unit must have established its superiority. All elite segments, by definition, must have a recognized claim to superiority in a branch of its profession. Such recognition of superiority results in prestige, an essential attribute of the elite. Finally, the Harvard physicians must be in positions to wield power to guide the decisions and practices of medicine.

The Harvard physicians making use of facilities at Boston City Hospital do share an understanding of the purposes of medicine. They share the academic rather than the traditional or more contemporary understanding of medicine. Their understanding is illustrated by Maxwell Finland, M.D., who as the head of the Harvard Medical Unit said:

> All teaching and research is oriented about the concept that the best care of the patient comes from the [knowledge] of his

chemical and physiological processes and their disturbances in disease, and that the management of the patient depends on a sympathetic application of this knowledge.[21]

In accord with such an understanding of the purposes of medicine, these physicians are most interested in the activity congenial to its implementation: research.

The Harvard physicians also agree that the proper attributes of a physician are clinical competence and scientific curiosity. The exemplary physician, to young men of the Harvard Medical Unit, is George R. Minot, M.D., 1934 Nobel Laureate in Medicine. He has been described as the "*Inquisitive Physician* whose penetrating inquiries into the minutiae of his patients' problems and close attention to details of the results of his ministrations earned him a Nobel award." [22] The rationale for the activity of these physicians is that a physician learns through concentrated attention to the effects of his treatment, and the patient benefits from the physician's new knowledge by receiving "a more rational application of therapy." [23] Accordingly, students, interns, and residents are encouraged to deal with a patient's illness as a disease entity and to learn how available remedies effect its course or cure.

The Harvard understanding of medicine is rooted in the bacteriologic period of medical history. In the late nineteenth century many disease-producing microorganisms were discovered, and research on their biology and physiology was established as a concern of medicine. At the same time disease began to be associated with bacteria, and advances were made in the clinical use of antibacterial substances. Discoveries and advances in bacteriology, pathology, and immunology in the

21. Maxwell Finland, M.D., is the George Richards Minot Professor of Medicine at the Harvard Medical School and Director of the Thorndike Memorial Laboratory and Second and Fourth (Harvard) Medical Services. This statement appeared in his report presented to the Faculty of Medicine, Harvard University, December 18, 1964.

22. Statement made by Maxwell Finland in "The Fruits of the Thorndike Memorial," *Harvard Medical Alumni Bulletin*, 39, 1 (Fall, 1964).

23. Finland, *Report of the Faculty of Medicine*, Harvard University, December 18, 1964.

early twentieth century were followed by new knowledge in nutrition and metabolism. Shepard and Roney have described this period as "the era of bacteriology and pathology."[24]

In 1923 the Thorndike Memorial Laboratory was established as a research facility in the tradition of the era. During the early years the clinical and research concerns of men at the Thorndike Laboratory were influenced by its first director, Francis W. Peabody, who had been on the staff of Peter Bent Brigham Hospital and had had both research and clinical experience at Rockefeller Hospital. After Peabody's death in 1927 the tradition was continued by George R. Minot, a physician trained in medicine and physiology, who became world famous for his research on the successful treatment of pernicious anemia. The work of men such as these illustrates the interest in research that has been characteristic of physicians at the Harvard Medical Unit since its establishment at Boston City Hospital.

As an affiliate of the Harvard Medical School, the Thorndike Laboratory, with the Second and Fourth Medical Services, shares in its prestige. But the Harvard Medical Unit has a reputation of its own—specifically for academic medicine. This reputation was established by physicians who successfully conducted basic studies of diseases and their management. In a recent assessment of advances in biochemistry, for example, only four were described as outstanding, of which three were the results of studies by physicians at the Thorndike Laboratory.[25] As pathbreakers in medicine, these men earned the Harvard Medical Unit prestige and at the same time established themselves as leaders in academic medicine.

24. William P. Shepard and James G. Roney, Jr., "The Teaching of Preventive Medicine in the United States," *Milbank Memorial Fund Quarterly*, XLII, 4 (October, 1964), Pt. 2, pp. 25–27.

25. Maxwell Finland, "The Training of the Physician," *The New England Journal of Medicine*, 271, 21 (November 19, 1964), p. 1097. The three advances in biochemical knowledge were "*thyroid-binding protein,* the functions of which were described and elucidated by Ingbar and Freinkel; *intrinsic factor,* a name synonymous with *Castle factor;* and *transferrin,* which was shown by Jandl and Katz to provide a sort of automatic cycle of doorstep delivery service of iron for hemoglobin production by the immature erythrocyte."

The prestige of an elite, however, depends only in part on reputation. It also requires power. As C. Wright Mills analyzed the conditions for elites:

> Some reputation must be mixed with power in order to create prestige. An elite cannot acquire prestige without power; it cannot retain prestige without reputation. Its past power and success build a reputation on which it can coast for a while. But it is no longer possible for the power of an elite based on reputation alone to be maintained against reputation that is based on power.[26]

A reputation without power would have given the Harvard Medical Unit no continuing prestige except that accrued from its affiliation with the Harvard Medical School. It would, of course, enjoy such esteem as society accords all physicians and medical institutions, but eventually its reputation within the medical world would lessen, and its physicians would no longer be unique in American medicine. Once the Harvard Medical Unit achieved its reputation, it was not difficult to obtain power.

The power of the Harvard Medical Unit is based on the policy of training young physicians for influential positions with other segments of the medical elite. For diverse reasons, established or promising physicians leave the Unit and continue their academic careers at other medical schools and affiliated institutions. Most of the physicians in the later stages of an academic career at Thorndike Laboratory are "maturing young investigators," who depend for support on research funds granted by the Public Health Service of the Department of Health, Education and Welfare. The limited number of tenured positions at the Harvard Medical School makes it impossible to tenure all the young men who might establish themselves in academic medicine. Many, finding themselves ready for senior appointments at a moment when none are available at the Harvard Medical Unit, move to other Harvard-affiliated groups of physicians or go to other medical schools. Leaving for better positions in the certainty that only circumstances prevented their staying,

26. C. Wright Mills, *The Power Elite* (New York, Oxford University Press, 1957), p. 88.

these men are not bitter, and a consciousness of fraternity persists.

The setting in which the Harvard Medical Unit exists fosters a fraternal spirit among the members of the medical services and research laboratories. As interns become involved with their work, for example, they have little contact with their counterparts elsewhere in the hospital. They do not so much lose contact with other versions of medicine as they become aware that they are somehow different. The distinctiveness of the Harvard Medical Unit becomes exaggerated. The far-from-perfect working conditions also promote a strong sense of identification with a distinguished society of good fellows, which persists long after they have left the Harvard Medical Unit.

Obviously, there are many such school-tie groups of physicians, but only a few others exert such nationwide influence on American medicine. The record is unique. From the Harvard Medical Unit have come twenty-eight deans of medical schools and numerous chairmen of departments at the "name" schools such as California, Illinois, Western Reserve, and Wisconsin. Many executives and members of the Association of American Physicians, the American Society for Clinical Investigation, and other select societies of academic medicine are also alumni of the Harvard Medical Unit.[27] Other alumni are on the American specialty boards, whose purpose is the "improvement of general standards of graduate medical education and facilities for special training."[28] At one time, five of the twelve members of the American Board of Internal Medicine had been either house officers or research fellows at Boston City Hospital. Two of the other seven members of that specialty board had trained at Harvard-affiliated Peter Bent Brigham Hospital.

27. Approximately 11 per cent of the active membership in 1963 of the Association of American Physicians and the American Society for Clinical Investigation had been at the Harvard Medical Unit. Also, "among the 61 members of the [then] newly organized Association of University Cardiologists, nine [were] present or past members of the Harvard Medical Unit at the Boston City Hospital." *Harvard Medical Alumni Bulletin,* 39, 1 (Fall, 1964).

28. "Policies of Approved Specialty Boards," *Directory of Medical Specialists* (Chicago, Marquis–Who's Who, Inc., 1963), p. 19, which is also the source of information on the educational histories of physicians.

The fact that physicians joining the Harvard Medical Unit come from "name" schools is *de facto* evidence of its status as a segment of the medical elite. Many, on leaving, also go to the top-flight institutions. That is, there are career moves between the Harvard group and other "name" groups of physicians. The reference to "name" schools is made without implication for quality. By 1960, fewer than twenty medical schools had produced more than 50 per cent of those on the medical staffs of American hospitals.[29] The "name" schools producing physicians of this sort include Harvard, which graduated 8.5 per cent of physicians on medical school faculties and 5 per cent of those with full-time hospital positions, Columbia, Johns Hopkins, Yale, Pennsylvania, Minnesota, Cornell, and Western Reserve.

Career moves to and from the Harvard Medical Unit are presented in Tables 3.1 and 3.2. In calculating the figures for Table 3.1, I have excluded all physicians awarded their M.D.s by any of the three Boston schools. The policy of the Harvard Medical Unit is to allocate half the number of intern positions to medical students entering from the graduating class of the Harvard Medical School. If the Harvard graduates who served as interns were included, 75 per cent of all the Harvard Medical Unit would have come from one of the "name" schools of medicine.

Many Harvard graduates wish to stay in Boston. As they well know, "The internship that a doctor serves is a distinctive badge [and] is one of the most enduring criteria in the evaluation of his status." [30] Physicians interning at Boston City Hospital may aspire to medical practice in the Boston metropolitan area. They might also go from the Harvard Medical Unit to Harvard-affiliated or other university groups of physicians in Boston. The physicians leaving to go to positions at the local medical schools were excluded from Table 3.2, with the intention of reflecting mobility between and not within medical systems.

All career moves between the Harvard Medical Unit and "name" schools of medicine are *prima facie* evidence of participation in the medical elite. Of all physicians who come to the

29. Oswald Hall, "The Stages of a Medical Career," p. 330.
30. Oswald Hall, "The Stages of a Medical Career."

Table 3.1. Academic Origins by Selected
"Name" Schools of Interns, Residents, and Other
Physicians at the Harvard Medical Unit

Medical school [a]	Number	Cumulative percentage
Columbia	35	9
Johns Hopkins	34	17
Cornell	18	22
California	17	26
Yale	16	30
Pennsylvania	16	34
Minnesota	14	38
Michigan	12	40
Washington U.	11	43
U. of Chicago	10	46
Western Reserve	9	48
Rochester	7	50
Total	199	50

[a] "Name" schools with five or more faculty members from the Harvard Unit at Boston City Hospital.
Source: Maxwell Finland, M.D.: also Table 1, *New England Journal of Medicine*, 271, 21 (November 19, 1964), p. 1097.

Harvard Medical Unit without a Harvard M.D., 50 per cent were from "name" schools.

Final evidence of the Harvard Medical Unit's elite status is the moves of its alumni to "name" schools. Good clinical experience is available at Boston City Hospital, and it would not be surprising to find physicians who, having obtained that experience and served an appropriate residency, go on to the private practice of a specialty. Many do just that. Others, however, go into academic medicine: One of every two physicians from the Harvard Medical Unit holds or has held an academic appointment in a medical school. Of those who do hold academic appointments, two of every five are at one of the "name" schools of American medicine. That is, 38 per cent have or had academic

Table 3.2. Career Moves to Selected "Name"
Schools by Alumni of the Harvard Medical Unit

Medical school [a]	Number	Cumulative percentage
Illinois	14	5
Western Reserve	14	9
Columbia	10	13
Minnesota	9	16
Cornell	8	18
California		
Los Angeles	7	20
San Francisco	7	23
Johns Hopkins	7	25
Wisconsin	7	27
Cincinnati	6	29
Pennsylvania	6	32
Yale	6	34
New York University	5	35
Rochester	5	37
Stanford	5	38
Total	116	38

[a] "Name" schools with five or more faculty members from the Harvard Medical Unit at Boston City Hospital.
Source: Maxwell Finland, M.D.; also Table, 5 *Harvard Medical Alumni Bulletin*, 39, 1 (Fall, 1964).

appointments at "name" medical schools. The others are distributed among some fifty other medical schools in America.

From the evidence, there is no doubt that the Harvard Medical Unit is not only a subculture of medicine but, in fact, a segment of the medical elite. Though it is only one segment, it is an important segment. Boston City Hospital makes available facilities and patients, and Harvard physicians make use of both to advance the purpose of their segment of the medical profession. Moreover, the Harvard segment controls many positions on the career ladder for its branch of the profession; that is, it can require medical school graduates who have academic aspirations to spend their time attending patients in exchange for the training and assistance necessary to obtain positions at medical schools. This, then, is the situation in which interns find themselves on the Harvard Medical Services at Boston City Hospital.

4. Candidates for the Medical Elite

To BE practicing physicians, all medical school graduates must serve an internship. This mandatory year may be spent at a city, county, community, or university hospital, in either a specialized or a rotating program of training. The kind of hospital an intern selects determines the patients he will see as well as the teaching he receives from practicing physicians. At community hospitals, for example, interns see private rather than house patients. They are taught by physicians in general or specialized practice, rather than by physicians teaching or conducting research at a medical school or affiliated medical setting. A specialized internship, no matter where it is served, provides considerable experience with patients whose medical problems are of particular interest to physicians in one of the medical specialties. The more typical specialized internships are internal medicine, surgery, pediatrics, obstetrics and gynecology, and pathology, the basic science of medicine. Rotating internships provide a variety of experiences, in all or a combination of the medical specialties.

Each kind of hospital and type of internship has a meaning of its own in the medical profession. Many physicians think it important for those who wish to specialize to begin their training early. Others think the practice of medicine is facilitated by comprehensive training and consider a rotating internship important for those who wish careers in private practice. No matter which internship he eventually selects, the student's decision at this point has implications for the kind of medical career he will have. In choosing one internship over another, students may turn their backs on some opportunities and commit themselves to others.

All medical students do not want the same kind of careers. Many want to be specialists but not scientists, or teachers; a few want to be general practitioners of medicine. Students are not passive spectators, but play a part in deciding what careers they will ultimately have by making decisions that affect the course of their training. Some may commit themselves as early as college by choosing premedical studies.[1] All who enter medical school are committed to medicine, but they commit themselves further when they choose their internships.[2] Obviously, students do not all choose the same kinds of internships. From among those internships available they pick the ones most in accord with their career aspirations.

The internships students serve result, in part, from the students' preference for one or another medical career. Yet there are well-planned efforts to steer them in particular directions. In order to survive, specialty groups, medical school faculties, group practices, every subgroup of physicians must have new members. This regeneration cannot be left to chance alone; all groups must evolve ways to recruit candidates. The Harvard Medical Unit is no exception; its survival depends on recruiting graduates who are not only willing to serve internships, but are in

1. Wagner Thielens, Jr., "Some Comparisons of Entrants to Medical and Law School," in Robert K. Merton and others, eds., *The Student Physician* (Cambridge, Harvard University Press for the Commonwealth Fund, 1957), pp. 131–152.
2. Patricia L. Kendall and Hanan C. Selvin, "Tendencies toward Specialization in Medical Training," in Merton, *The Student Physician*, pp. 153–174.

fact potential candidates for careers as scientists and teachers of medicine. A year in which all its interns planned to become general practitioners would be calamitous, since they would enter practice immediately after the mandatory year of training, leaving the Unit with no qualified candidates for assistant residencies. In other words, the Harvard Medical Unit would not have the people it needs to occupy its positions and thereby maintain itself at Boston City Hospital. The Unit has therefore developed procedures to recruit interns who are at least considering careers as specialists, teachers, or scientists.

The graduates of almost any medical school could serve the Harvard internships at Boston City Hospital. Today, one can get a good medical education at all medical schools, and it seems likely that any student who had done well could manage an intern's job. "The bottom of a Harvard class may be better than the bottom of a class at some other school," explained a senior resident, "but the top of the class at most schools is just as good as the top of a Harvard class and could do the job at The City." But would the graduates of any medical school be candidates for careers as specialists, teachers, and scientists? Needless to say, the answer is that they would not. Many graduates want nothing more than to be able to begin medical practice. How, then, does the Harvard Medical Unit assure itself a sufficient number of students who aspire to the elite careers of medicine?

THE PORTS OF ENTRY FOR THE MEDICAL ELITE

As there are "name" medical schools, so are there "name" internships. Most of the former are familiar to the American public, but few of the internships are at all well known. Those that may be recognized are affiliated with "name" schools or at such "name" hospitals as the Massachusetts General in Boston or Bellevue in New York City. Although the layman may know the names of medical schools and hospitals operating programs for the training of physicians, he knows little and probably cares less about the specific internships and residencies that make up graduate medical education in America.

The Second and Fourth (Harvard) Medical Services at Boston City Hospital are noted for producing academic physicians. Medical school students who aspire to academic careers are therefore advised by faculty members and other physicians to serve their internships there:

> Several members of our faculty have trained [at the Harvard Medical Services]; others were acquainted with it through friendships with men who had trained there. I spoke to several faculty members about it and wrote the BCH for information. I was advised by several faculty members that BCH was a fine place to intern [and] I am told that after finishing my training at BCH I can go anywhere and do anything.[3]

Medical students who choose university internships like Harvard's seek careers as specialists, scientists, teachers, or some combination of academic activities and specialty practice. One wrote, "I want to teach and perhaps do research part-time, combining practice with teaching, and if I become interested in a worthwhile problem, devoting time to research." Another said, "I want to be on the faculty of a good medical school; some time teaching, quite a bit of research, a few private patients." By their choice of internship, they announce their candidacy for this kind of career. Almost all interns at the Harvard Medical Services have more or less turned their backs on the general practice of medicine. "I would like a general practice," wrote only one of the sixteen medical students accepted in 1965, "being well qualified in all major areas, that is, medicine, surgery, pediatrics and OB-GYN, [but] I'm constantly told this is impractical." The Harvard internships are not the kind one serves only to meet the requirements for a license to practice medicine. The fact is made obvious by the following comments of a senior resident:

> I asked the senior resident, "What are you looking for in an applicant to the Harvard Medical Services?" He answered, "Well, let me first point out that interviews here do not carry

3. All incoming interns at the Harvard Medical Service in 1965–1966 were required to complete a questionnaire before they arrived. See Appendix II. The comments attributed to medical students in this section were, unless indicated, from that questionnaire or accompanying correspondence.

a great deal of weight, and people are accepted or rejected mostly in terms of where they stood in their medical school class and the kind of recommendations they get. But I suppose, in general, what we look for in the interview is some assurance that the fellow is reasonably mature and sensible. The people coming here obviously are all intelligent. We look for what their interests in the future might be. I think, by and large, people coming here are interested in academic careers, and somebody who is interested in general practice in Rudolph Junction, probably, this isn't the internship for him."

"Let's say a fellow came to you," I said; "let's say I came to you standing high in my class at medical school, and I have three decent recommendations, my Dean says I'm going to be a great doctor but a practicing physician, and I definitely am not going into academic medicine. How would this weigh?"

The senior resident, shaking his head, explained, "It would probably weigh against you. I've never been in on the final acceptance or rejection of interns [but] I would think that they would tend to be rejected if they were definitely going into practice, unless they were extraordinary people."

The Harvard program of graduate medical training is more than just simply a way to meet licensing requirements; the Harvard Medical Services are a "name"—a port of entry for the medical elite. By 1964, 873 medical school graduates had served as interns, residents, research fellows, and staff members of the Harvard Medical Unit at Boston City Hospital. A brief consideration of their subsequent careers establishes the Unit as one of the places where routes to careers in academic medicine begin. As Maxwell Finland wrote:

> We have nearly arrived at the half-century mark of the firm establishment of the Harvard affiliation of the Fourth Medical Service and the 40th anniversary of the Thorndike Memorial Laboratory. . . . I had occasion to review the attainments of the alumni of the [Boston City] Hospital and could not help but be impressed by the extraordinarily large number of them, particularly those of the Harvard Medical Unit, who have become leaders in academic medicine.[4]

4. Maxwell Finland, "The Fruits of the Thorndike Memorial," *Harvard Medical Alumni Bulletin*, 39, 1 (Fall, 1964).

Table 4.1. Medical Schools at which Harvard Medical Unit Alumni Hold Positions as Assistant Professors, Associate Professors, and Professors

Medical school	Number of academic appointments	Percentage of academic appointments
City of Boston:		
Harvard University	57	15
Tufts University	18	4
Boston University	17	4
National "Name":		
16 schools of medicine	122	32
National "Other":		
57 schools of medicine	173	45
Total	387	100

Source: Table 5, "The Fruits of the Thorndike Memorial," *Harvard Medical Alumni Bulletin,* 39, 1 (Fall, 1964).

Table 4.1 presents the positions at medical schools attained by these "leaders in academic medicine." A significant number of those who began their medical careers at the Harvard Medical Unit do, in fact, continue in academic medicine. Of those who began at the Harvard Medical Unit, a few more than 11 per cent attained positions as professors; almost 16 per cent became associate professors; and another 12 per cent were assistant professors at schools of medicine. A significant number of those who began their careers at other places but continued them at Harvard Medical Unit also held positions in academic medicine. Of these, 25 per cent were professors; 17 per cent were associate professors; and another 13 per cent were assistant professors at schools of medicine.

Not all career routes that began at the Harvard Medical Unit led to the Harvard Medical School. They led to academic appointments in American medicine generally. Of those who have or had academic appointments, approximately one in five were at one of the three Boston medical schools. More than 75 per cent of those who had been interns or residents held at one time or another academic positions at 73 other medical schools in the United States. In other words, an internship served at the Harvard Medical Unit usually leads to an academic position of some sort at a medical school. Thus the Harvard Medical Unit is not only an elite segment but is also a port of entry for those aspiring to academic careers. The training one gets there permits progress toward academic positions, and those recruited for that training are on their way to the first rung of the ladder of an elite career in medicine.

Sociologists are concerned with the origins of members of the groups they study. For my purpose, it is the academic rather than the social origin that is important. Medical students applying for internships could come from any of more than a hundred medical schools. The faculties at those schools do not all agree on what medicine is and place different values on the activities around which physicians could organize their careers. When selecting medical students who would be most qualified as interns, members of any particular segment would prefer those whose understanding of medicine is compatible with their own. Academic origins are relevant variables of recruitment, because the kinds of training candidates have had is differentially valued by the various segments of the profession. For the medical elite, internship candidates from schools known for training general practitioners are less desirable than graduates of schools with reputations for teaching and research.

Does a viable elite group select only the graduates of "name" medical schools for internships? If not, are there other routes that afford access to persons from the less prestigious schools? More specifically, from which medical schools are interns selected, and why are they chosen, to begin their careers at the Harvard Medical Unit? [5]

If only a few "name" schools did, in fact, provide all the personnel for elite groups of physicians, then the medical elite would be a relatively uncomplicated social phenomenon—merely

5. This question is a paraphrase of one asked about social origins as part of a study of American chemists. Anselm L. Strauss and Lee Rainwater, *The Professional Scientist* (Chicago, Aldine, 1962), p. 53.

a stratum of the medical profession comprising "name" schools of equal reputation, with personnel whose knowledge and skills were superior to those at other schools of medicine. Any stratum of medicine would be no more than an association of medical schools having a common reputation and physicians who share the same or similar understandings of medicine. If, on the other hand, the "name" schools provide most, but not all, personnel for a group of the medical elite, then other factors must influence the selection of candidates for elite careers.

Fifty per cent of all those serving internships on the Second and Fourth Medical Services during the study were graduates of the Harvard Medical School (see Table 4.2). Another 30 per cent were from "name" schools like Cornell, Yale, Johns Hopkins, and Minnesota. But the remaining 20 per cent came from other medical schools, such as Utah, Florida, Illinois, and the recently established Seton Hall in Jersey City, New Jersey. Furthermore, of those who went on to become assistant residents, 16 per cent were from other than "name" schools. Of those from American schools who traveled the entire route to the staff of the Thorndike Laboratory and a Harvard Medical School appointment, one in seven were not from "name" schools. Thus, though only a few do so, it is possible for a graduate of a less celebrated medical school to begin his career with an internship on the Harvard Medical Services and progress to an academic appointment at Harvard Medical School or some other school of medicine.

Since not all candidates for the elite come from "name" schools, some other variable must influence their selection. I cannot demonstrate conclusively that what is operating is the recruiting mechanism by which elite groups maintain themselves within the profession, though I strongly suggest that this is so. Physician groups use medical education to attract candidates. "The medical school curriculum today is crowded as the medical specialties compete for the student's time and attention, seeking to recruit or at least to socialize the budding professional into the correct attitudes toward [specialty groups]." [6]

Each group of physicians must compete with other groups for

6. Rue Bucher and Anselm Strauss, "Professions in Process," *American Journal of Sociology*, LXVI (January, 1961), p. 331.

Table 4.2. Academic Origins of Interns and Assistant Residents on the Harvard Medical Services at Boston City Hospital, July 1, 1963–June 30, 1966

Medical school awarding M.D.	Total Interns	Total Assistant residents	Per cent Interns	Per cent Assistant residents
Harvard	24	16	50	37
"Name" Schools	15	20	31	47
Other	9	7	19	16
Total	48	43	100	100

candidates for its careers. All groups attempt to gain some control of the recruitment process and to guarantee that a sufficient number of candidates select their particular segment. There are not enough "name" medical school graduates for all the internships that launch elite careers. Also, physicians at medical schools share the aversion to inbreeding characteristic of almost all of academia. This further reduces the number of candidates by setting a limit on the number of graduates of a given medical school to serve its own internships. The Harvard Medical Unit, for example, limits the number of Harvard Medical School graduates to eight, half the internships it offers at Boston City Hospital. Graduates of other schools, then, must be recruited, and if candidates from "name" schools are not available, recruiters must turn to other schools.

My first hint of a recruiting policy came during my first few days at Boston City Hospital. At a meeting of the Harvard Medical Society, when discussing the academic attainment of physicians who began or continued their careers at the Harvard Medical Unit, Maxwell Finland told his colleagues:

> All told, the professors have been spread among 76 of the medical schools and 3 colleges in this country and among 30 medical schools in foreign lands. The "colonization" of certain

of these schools by former members of the Harvard Medical Unit (and some also from other Harvard-affiliated Units) of the Boston City Hospital is an interesting subject in itself, but not for here.[7]

There is no difficulty in documenting that the Harvard Medical Unit has colonized certain medical schools. A number of schools have an unusually large number of professors who are alumni of the Unit, either attracted to those schools by former members of the Unit or sent by those schools to be trained by Harvard physicians. At Western Reserve, for example, there was an effort to recruit the Unit's alumni and fourteen physicians from the Unit have been appointed to the faculty of Western Reserve Medical School. These physicians are a *de facto* colony.

Medical school colonization of this sort obviously has implications for recruitment by the Unit. They are not, however, the obvious implications. When I first became aware of colonization, for example, my hypothesis was that the Unit attempted to place its alumni at "name" schools so that they could recruit students for internships at Boston City Hospital. The following excerpt from my notes demonstrates that this is not so:

> Brahm began by explaining to me how interns were selected. The approximate number of applicants, his best guess, is 260; approximately 70 from Harvard. He made it quite clear that these were his opinions. The policy, he stated, was to select a group of interns, half of whom were from Harvard and half from other medical schools. Interns, he said, are selected on the basis of academic record and letters of recommendation. When I asked which played a greater part in the selection of interns—acedemic record or letters of recommendation—he said, "It's mostly their class standing."
>
> I presented a hypothetical case: a boy from Seton Hall in the top 10 per cent of his class and a boy from the University of Minnesota in the top 10 per cent of his class; both apply for internships at the Harvard Medical Unit. How would you choose between the two applicants? The hypothetical case was

7. Maxwell Finland in the *Harvard Medical Alumni Bulletin*, 39, 1 (Fall, 1964). I first heard recruitment and colonization discussed on the Medical Services on April 14, 1964.

a bad one, because they had just selected a boy from Seton Hall Medical School. But it did get him talking about "getting into Harvard."

Brahm then explained that it was not only class standing but what school the applicant was from. Also, his letters of recommendation were important. If they came from people who were either graduates of Harvard, students of professors at Harvard, or known by professors at Harvard, they would help his application. This, he thought, played a greater part in the selection of interns than the physicians of the Harvard Medical Unit would admit. [April 14, 1964]

In this discussion I contrasted Seton Hall Medical School to the University of Minnesota because Seton Hall had only recently been established. My assumption was that no candidate for an elite career would have come from a medical school established less than a decade ago. The assumption was wrong. One other intern was from Georgetown University. I was somewhat surprised that Catholic medical schools contributed two of the sixteen interns for 1964, but the academic origins of the others were in no way surprising.

The following comments by Maxwell Finland describe the conditions that resulted in, among others, a career route from Seton Hall to the Harvard Medical Unit:

In this country several schools have an unusually large number of professors who are alumni of the Harvard Medical Unit at the Boston City Hospital, either attracted there by former members of the Unit or selected by the latter for training at City Hospital. Thus, Dr. Joseph T. Wearn attracted a number of bright and promising young men from this unit after he left it to head the Department of Medicine at Western Reserve. Dr. Chester S. Keefer got most of his original staff from among members of this unit when he left to accept the Chair of Medicine at Boston University. Most of the professors from this unit who are at the University of Illinois were attracted there by Dr. Harry F. Dowling, who received some of his early training at the Thorndike. Dr. Harold Jeghers, an intimate friend and admirer, though not an alumnus, of the Harvard Medical Unit, sent some of his staff here for training and attracted others from there to join him when he became head of the Department of Medicine at Seton Hall.[8]

Our schools of medicine contain "colonies" of physicians who belong to the same medical fellowship. As I have noted, physicians leaving the Harvard Medical Unit continue to identify with one another as alumni of Harvard at Boston City Hospital. Many of those who leave for positions at other medical schools have been told throughout their careers that they will be members of a select group. Graduates of "name" schools are told from the beginning of their careers that they are the select of the medical profession. For example, at the 1965 dinner of the Harvard Medical Alumni Association, new graduates heard: "I welcome you; not into the Great Society sponsored by a rival organization, but into the Most Exclusive Society in this country—the Harvard Medical Alumni Association."[9] A similar scene is repeated, with only slight variation, at most "name" schools of American medicine. For those physicians, the fellowship of Harvard Medical Unit alumni is nothing less than they expect: membership in an elite.

Not all physicians continue to be members of elite Harvard units. Some physicians have to leave Harvard; but they realize that the circumstances of their going have nothing to do with them personally, and they require no "cooling."[10] That is, those who leave do so without a feeling of failure that would end their relationship with the Harvard Medical Unit. As a physician who was considering a better position than he had or could anticipate if he stayed said: "All of us are good, but there just aren't enough slots for all the good men that want to stay." Thus those who go continue to consider themselves part of the physician group at Boston City Hospital. They are the "bird dogs" who recruit promising candidates for the Harvard Medical Unit.

8. Maxwell Finland, "The Training of the Physician," *New England Journal of Medicine*, 271, 21 (November 19, 1964), p. 1099.

9. Langdon Parsons, Harvard '27, at the Alumni Council Dinner, March 8, 1965.

10. Erving Goffman, "On Cooling the Mark Out: Some Aspects of Adaptation to Failure," *Psychiatry*, 15 (November, 1952), pp. 451–463.

For example, eleven alumni of the unit were on the faculty of Seton Hall and played no small part in the recruitment of that school's graduates.

Recruitment for this segment of the elite is accomplished by a network of "bird dog" colonies of physicians who owe allegiance to the Harvard Medical Unit. This procedure, for lack of any better label, I call the colonial policy of the medical elite.[11] The medical schools with three or more faculty members who had interned at the Harvard Medical Services accounted for 20 per cent of incoming interns. There were approximately 50 such alumni at half a dozen schools. The statistic becomes significant when compared to the 6 per cent who came from almost 60 other schools, at which 185 other alumni held academic positions. The implication is that a function of the alumni contingents is to contribute personnel to the parent group. The number of those serving internships during the years in which the study was conducted is small, but the proportion of those graduating from "colony" schools makes tenable the hypothesis that recruiting for the medical elite is accomplished by a network of career routes from "name" schools and other less celebrated schools that have been colonized by alumni of the Harvard Medical Unit.

Since the model for elite recruitment evolved from data obtained during field work in 1964, I could obtain additional documentation only from those who were serving Harvard internships in 1965. In that year, eight interns were from other than "name" schools of medicine. The relevant circumstances of their choice of internship are summarized in Table 4.3. Six of the eight learned of the program from members of the faculty at their own medical schools. Five of these six reported having discussed the choice of an internship with at least three faculty members who had been at the Harvard Medical Unit. Although they learned of the internships and were advised to apply for it, only two of the six thought their decision to do so had been influ-

11. A colony is either a school identified as such by physicians of the Harvard Medical Unit or one having three or more alumni reported by those beginning careers in 1965 to have influenced their decisions to choose Boston City Hospital.

Table 4.3. Questions Regarding Decisions to Seek Internship Appointments at the Harvard Medical Unit and Responses of Medical Students Selected from Other Than "Name" Medical Schools to Begin Careers at Boston City Hospital in 1965.

Questions	Number
How did you learn about the internship program at Boston City Hospital?	
From a member of my medical school faculty	6
From a friend now at the Harvard Medical Services	2
Do you know if any of your medical school faculty had been at Boston City Hospital?	
Yes, many	2
Yes, one of the largest contingents	1
Yes, at least 3 had	5
Did any particular person influence your decision to intern at Boston City Hospital?	
No	3
Internship adviser	1
Faculty members who had been there	2
Friend who had been there	2
Were you advised to intern at Boston City Hospital?	
Yes, by faculty members who had been there	6
No	2

Source: Questionnaire completed by medical students prior to beginning at Boston City Hospital. See Appendix II.

enced by faculty members who were Harvard Medical Unit alumni. Medical school graduates beginning careers may not be aware of the role Harvard Medical Unit alumni have played in their coming to Boston City Hospital. Graduates of the other than "name" schools who are further along the career routes talk freely about the circumstances of recruitment and sponsorship; also, they have learned a great deal about routes to careers within the Harvard Medical Unit.

I asked, "You did have a couple of men [your medical school] who had been at Boston City Hospital, no?" He nodded his head and replied, "I don't kid myself; [my medical school] is small and my references were important . . . the Dean and some faculty people had been at Boston City Hospital." He told me that he had heard about the internship from faculty who had been at the hospital for training. After finishing his assistant residency, he wants to stay on at the Thorndike.

I asked, "How much do you think you improved your chances of working with [a 'great' man at the Thorndike] by serving a Boston City Hospital internship?" He replied, "I would say infinitely. I mean, just the fact that you've been here. I think this group takes care of its own . . . Senior residents are invariably people who have been assistant residents here [and] people who have done their training here from time immemorial have been the people that end up being chief resident. Those people who really express a desire usually get a job if they have not messed up or unless they haven't really done good jobs [as interns]." (December 15, 1964)

All of those from lesser-known schools who chose the Harvard Medical Unit program in 1965 were graduates of medical schools where Harvard alumni constituted a colony. Most learned about the program from, discussed it with, and were advised to choose it by Harvard Medical Unit alumni.

THE ASPIRATIONS OF CANDIDATES FOR ELITE MEDICAL CAREERS

Sociological studies have usually assumed that the choice of an internship is a result of career aspiration. Different career goals will determine what is and what is not important about the internships. The choices of students at any one medical school, however, will be varied, because all students seldom have the same aspirations. There is little homogeneity of aspiration in medical schools, as measured by students' choice of internships. A study of the University of Kansas Medical School, for example, demonstrated that the criteria for judging internships were intelligible to all students, but that the students disagreed on the relative importance of particular criteria. Sociologists conducting the Kansas study reported:

In making [internship] choices students make use of certain collective understandings about the nature of an internship and the advantages one might gain from one. Further, these collective understandings define the particular advantages and disadvantages associated with each kind of internship. These understandings do not, however, specify which kind of internship one should desire or choose, for students recognize that individual students may have different views of what will be important for them to get out of their internship.[12]

Theoretically, there should be homogeneity of aspiration among students who choose to serve the same kind of internships. I will document that students choosing Harvard internships at Boston City Hospital do share similar hopes.

Students most often choose a number of internships; during the fourth year of medical school they apply for various ones, listing their order of preference. Applicants are in turn ranked by the groups to which they apply. Students' lists of internships are matched to physicians' lists of students. Each year this national matching program brings together students and the hospitals at which they will intern. Let us consider the other choices of interns at the Harvard Medical Unit. If they chose the same or similar programs, we could conclude that there was a collective aspiration characteristic of those beginning on routes to elite medical careers.

Table 4.4 lists the other internship programs chosen by the 1965 Harvard Medical Unit interns. All 61 had applied to more than 29 programs in the United States. In six cases the choice was based on geographical proximity to the students' homes. If we exclude these, our group considered only 22 other internships. Excluding all other Harvard internships, we reduce the number of alternative choices to fewer than 20. The group's agreement concerning available programs is further illustrated by the fact that three out of four applied to the same 12 programs. Besides the Harvard internship programs at the Massachusetts General, Peter Bent Brigham, and Beth Israel hospitals, 12 of the 16 had applied to at least one of the internship programs affiliated with the following medical schools: Western Reserve, Minnesota,

12. Howard S. Becker and others, *Boys in White* (Chicago, University of Chicago Press, 1961), p. 385.

Table 4.4. Other Internship Choices of Interns Beginning on the Harvard Medical Services in 1965 Compared to the Choices of the Harvard Medical School Classes of 1962 and 1964

Medical school or hospital	Harvard Medical Unit 1965	Harvard Medical School [a] Class of 1962	Class of 1964
Harvard	18	18	17
Massachusetts General Hospital	7	7	7
Peter Bent Brigham Hospital	5	6	6
Beth Israel Hospital	6	5	4
Western Reserve	5	2	3
Minnesota	4	4	3
Washington U. (Barnes Hospital)	4	1	1
Cornell (New York Hospiatl)	5	1	0
Yale	5	0	0
U. of Washington	0	0	2
Columbia	3	0	3
Duke	2	2	0
Johns Hopkins	2	1	0
California	2	1	4
Strong Memorial Hospital, Rochester, N.Y.	2	1	0
Pennsylvania	1	0	0
North Carolina	2	1	0
Vanderbilt	1	0	1
Utah	1	1	0
Bronx Municipal Hospital Center, NYC	4	0	2
New York University	2	1	1
King County, Seattle	4	1	1
Cleveland Metropolitan General Hospital	3	1	1
Buffalo General Hospital	2	1	6
Other	5	7	13

[a] Only those graduates who entered straight internships in medicine; rotating and surgical internships were excluded to make the internship choices comparable to the programs entered by graduates of Harvard Medical School.

Washington (St. Louis), New York Hospital (Cornell), Yale, King County (Seattle), and the Bronx Municipal Hospital. Comparing the choices listed in Table 4.5 to the internships

Table 4.5 Career Aspirations of Those Serving Internships on the Harvard Medical Services in 1964 and 1965

Kind of medical school awarding M.D.	Career plans				
	General practice	Specialty practice	Research and/or teaching	Undecided	Total
"Name"	0	6	15	1	22
Other	1	1	6	2	10
Total	1	7	21	3	32

obtained by students at the Harvard Medical School, we see that the internships chosen are typical of those applied for by students at "name" schools of medicine. Choices of Harvard Medical Unit interns who had been students at "name" schools did not differ significantly from those of students who had graduated from other schools of medicine. No matter what their school of origin, the interns who came to the Harvard Medical Unit chose not only the same kind of program, a straight medical one, but selected internships at the same hospitals.

On the basis of data regarding internship choices in 1964, we may conclude that those who came to the Harvard Medical Unit had similar aspirations and agreed on the kinds of internships that were "good" and the places at which to serve them.

When contacted during the fourth year of medical school, most students who chose Harvard internships at Boston City Hospital reported that they had sought alternatives to the traditional medical practice and had been considering careers as specialists, scientists, or teachers, or a combination of all three. With only one exception, they had decided against general practice. Specialty practice was only slightly more attractive to them. The career aspirations of Harvard interns in 1964 and 1965 are presented in Table 4.5. Most interns apparently chose Harvard internships because of elite aspirations; they wanted careers as scientists and teachers more than any of the other careers in medicine. Since most students say they want those careers and a majority do, in fact, eventually have them, there can be little argument that there is a relationship between aspirations and the course of travel toward medical careers. Logically, people with specific career aspirations will more often attempt to gain access to and advance along the routes to those careers than will people without those aspirations.

During the early weeks of the internship year, interns were asked which careers they wanted for themselves. When explaining their preferences, they were most often vague and noncommittal. The following example illustrates the generalities with which they described their elite aspirations:

> I think an ideal medical career would be one in which an individual was happy and a service to medicine as well as his community. I think this could be done by going into academic medicine in a specialty and devoting time to teaching, research, and patients. In this way, you will contribute in many ways to the advancement of medicine while at the same time leading a respectable, rewarding, and comfortable personal life. [July 1, 1965]

All students agreed that a Harvard internship or one like it would advance their careers. Exactly what kind of career they were advancing toward was explained only by the term "academic medicine." For them, the future was some still-to-be-determined combination of teaching, research, and possibly a limited practice located in a university-affiliated medical setting rather than the usual doctor's office. As we shall see, the aspirations of Harvard interns prescribed the specific action necessary to advance toward a worthwhile career but left nebulous the activities that would constitute their future careers.

Additional data obtained from medical students further documented the general character of the aspirations that influenced their choice of internship. Most of them did not exclude any of the activities of medicine; they said they would like to do a little of everything—teaching, research, and caring for patients. Their aspirations did not change significantly during the course of the internship year. In the following excerpt from field notes, an intern at the end of his year described the future he wanted as a physician:

> I was with Brahm and we were discussing what he had learned during the year . . . I asked why he decided to serve his internship at Boston City Hospital. He said, "Well, because it has an excellent faculty, a very excellent group of people, and I wanted to have something to do with them, and the fact that I'm going into academic medicine and wanted an internship which . . . you know, looks good on paper."
> I said, "You said at lunch that you'll go anywhere you can get a good job. What is a good job?" Brahm said, "Not in order of importance: financial security," he laughed, "it would be in order, an institution where they give me what I want, and that is the opportunity to teach, hopefully, good students, not mediocre students. Also, the opportunity to do research, and a chance to practice a little bit of medicine." "But," I asked, "don't you want a practice?" He shook his head and said, "I don't want to have a private practice. I'd like to have private patients whom I'd see because they were referred to me, but no practice." [May 24, 1965]

Interns admit that they have chosen the Harvard Medical Unit because the demands of practice dissuade them from traditional medical careers. Students, interns, and residents all agree that a physician should serve, but they also know that being of service as a practitioner will require arranging their lives around the problems of maintaining a practice and the demands of patients. The following excerpt from my field notes illustrates the thinking of those students who look toward alternatives to careers as practitioners:

> Condon [assistant resident], who was sitting with Walters [visiting physician], waved to me and I moved over to join them. They were only a few chairs away from us at the same table. Walters was in practice and telling Condon about a

patient he had. He is an alumnus of the Harvard Medical Unit and practices in Boston. When he finished telling his story he looked at his watch, nodded, and got up to leave the dining hall. Condon turned to me and said, "I'd like to go into practice too, but I'm afraid the patients would kill me."

I at first thought he meant his attitude toward patients would get him into trouble. I asked what he meant, and he said: "In my home town we've got about 15,000 people. In the county, I guess, about 45,000 people. In the town there are about ten doctors there who care for these people. That's a big, demanding practice." I asked how practice was demanding. He said, "Well, Walters has to go out in the middle of the night. His patients think he's making all kinds of money when he really isn't getting rich. Like this patient he was telling us about. There are four of them working on the case, special nurses around the clock, labs, equipment, and the hospital and all. It's a $9,000 hospital bill. That's the cost of the medical care. He said they agreed they're not taking a fee and don't expect one, but after it's all over, those people will say I had a $9,000 hospital bill. That's the cost of medical care. You have to put up with that and that attitude toward the doctor too."

I asked what else you had to put up with in practice and he said, "You can't have a regular family life and you die at a young age. That's what I meant by patients killing me. The demands they make age you quickly. Walters will be an old man by 50; he didn't get started till he was about 32; he really won't have a long life."

I asked him what his future plans were. He said, "After I finish at NIH, I'll probably come back here to Thorndike. I'd like to have a few patients, but not really a practice. I think academic medicine will give me a chance to have a normal family life and not make the demands which would make me an old man before my time. With a few patients, I could be called on to consult or advise and still do my work. I hope to be able to get a good appointment at some university when I finish my residency. I hope to do enough to get such an appointment." [November 17, 1964]

All interns at one time or another spoke of having a future career similar to that described as "ideal" by the medical school graduate beginning his internship, or "good" by the intern completing his year at Boston City Hospital. They know it is not solely a medical practice they want, but a chance "to practice a little bit of medicine." They prefer nothing more than "the opportunity to do research." This aspiration and the way it must be fulfilled is illustrated by the following conversation with a medical student who gained his clinical experience on the Harvard Medical Services and applied for an internship at Boston City Hospital:

> I asked, "Would it be fair to say that you go to the Harvard Medical Unit if you want to go into academic medicine?"
>
> He replied, "No, if you want the opportunity to go into academic medicine you would go to a place like that, and if you find you don't want to go into academic medicine, you can always practice. In going to a place like the Harvard-Medical Unit you more or less avoid making that decision—academic or practice? In other words, you can sit around and wait for openings. If you remain long enough at The City, who knows what'll happen. There is a sudden possibility, doors open, or something of that sort will happen. You don't know how things will go. If you're not in a position to know, you won't have the opportunity." [January 20, 1965]

In general, Harvard interns want careers other than those ordinarily available to medical school graduates. They want to be something besides practicing physicians. They do not know exactly what it is they will do in the future, but they do know that serving internships like these will give them many possibilities and put them in a position to take advantage of opportunity when it does present itself. One intern on the Second Medical Service explained: "There are probably other places that have as good teachers and the same type of patients that this place does, [but] because it was a possibility that I would want to go into academic medicine and since one ought not cut one's own throat, I chose the Boston City Hospital." [13]

Not knowing exactly which careers they want, but knowing they should not close any doors, medical students interested in something besides practice choose internships that afford maxi-

13. *Intern,* June 11, 1965.

mum opportunities rather than those that commit them to specific career routes. It may well be that those who do not obtain internships at, let us say, Massachusetts General Hospital, feel that their careers have been damaged because they have fewer alternatives to becoming practicing physicians.

Medical students who said they wanted to become scientists and teachers did move toward those goals through their Harvard internships at Boston City Hospital, but they were not necessarily committed to these careers. The aspirations of the Harvard interns encompass elite careers, but not exclusively. Contrary to what one might expect, students' choices of internships result as much from their desire to remain uncommitted as from particular elite aspirations.

With respect to specific activities of medicine, these interns' ambitions are broad, encompassing all but general practice. In fact, what they all aspire to is some alternative to traditional medicine. They share a desire to make no specific commitments that would preclude taking advantage of any and all opportunities that could lead to a worthwhile medical career. They do not know what their opportunities will be, but they do know that this particular internship or one like it will put them in a position to choose among many attractive alternatives. This kind of thinking, rather than any specific elite aspiration, is what influences students to choose the Harvard Medical Unit.

THE CRITERIA FOR JUDGING INTERNSHIPS

The career aspirations of medical students are translated into immediate perspectives on internships. To make the actual choice students employ criteria that are in accord with their aspirations and their understanding of the actions necessary to obtain the careers they want. As their aspirations were homogeneous, so students who came to the Harvard Medical Unit in 1965 agreed on what was and what was not important to consider in choosing internships. Their criteria are presented in Table 4.6. Of the seven cited, the first criterion was geographic location. A few interns had thought it was not an important consideration. Six of the nine who thought location important had applied for at

Table 4.6. Criteria for Judging Internships Chosen by Interns Beginning on the Harvard Medical Services in 1965

Level of criteria	Criterion	Important? Yes	No	Typical comments [a]
Career	Location	9	7	"Either New York or Boston" "Boston is tops in medicine"
	Prestige	15	0	"Better chance of a good residency" "I plan a career in academic medicine"
	Professional Contacts	13	2	"It'll be a pleasure to meet some of the men I've heard about" "I want to stay in Boston, so a hospital here is good for my career"
Clinical Experience	Responsibility	16	0	"Want a great deal of it" "Get a great deal"
	Patients	12	3	"Get only house cases, so you have the responsibility" "A heavy load of acutely ill patients"
	Teaching	16	0	"Outstanding" "Good advice and up-to-date ideas when you want them"
	Facilities and Working Conditions	8	7	"They are poor and argue against going to Boston City Hospital" "You must ignore when applying to Boston City Hospital"

[a] Comments offered by interns in explanation of the criteria they nployed in judging Boston City Hospital.

least one internship close to communities where they had family and, if they were unable to obtain an elite position, would want to establish a practice. Location also matters to students who want to stay or locate in Boston:

I am a Bostonian and will remain a Bostonian, or put it this way: If I get a Boston internship, I'll probably be buried here. I have an interest in remaining and remaining on their terms. Since I want to remain in the Harvard group, I don't want to go into exile, and this is sort of what happens if you don't have connections at the Harvard hospitals. [January 20, 1965]

The location of an internship determines with which urban system of medical institutions and what group of physicians the candidates become associated. Those who wish nothing more than to establish a general practice of medicine choose internships located in the communities where they hope to practice. Similarly, students who want other careers choose internships that will involve them in those particular urban spheres where their interests are best represented. Specialists, scientists, and teachers are generally trained in Chicago, New York, or Boston; where they intern, however, will more or less determine where they take up their work. Location is also important because it leads to friendships and connections that will enhance a career. Interning in the community where he hopes to settle will facilitate a physician's efforts to build a practice. Similarly, the location of a university internship will facilitate an academic career in a particular urban sphere of medicine.

A second criterion may explain why location is less important for those seeking academic careers than for those who plan to establish medical practices: All Harvard Medical Unit interns agreed that prestige was an important consideration in choosing an internship. The prestige of a particular training program is something that can be taken from city to city. Some internships may be so well known that they serve as credentials for entry into the academic circles of any other urban sphere of the medical profession. One intern, for example, explained that he chose a Harvard internship because of his desire to enter academic medicine in another city.

I asked, "Since you knew you would be going back to be a resident, why did you come to BCH?" Roget said, "I had a friend in medical school, a very good friend who was here two years ago as an intern. Of course, I heard it was a good place but I took my cue from him. The other reason was that

I wanted to come to Boston. I feel I went to an excellent
medical schoool, but I wanted to get away for a year. I'm
going back, but I wanted to come to Harvard."

I asked him why, and he explained, "Well, because it is an
excellent faculty; a very excellent group of people, and I
wanted to have something to do with them. I'm going into
academic medicine, and I wanted the internship which was
the best or very good, I think of the word 'prestige,' a great
deal of prestige in being part of this group. It just has a very
very good reputation, you know. It will look good on paper."
[May 24, 1965]

When senior residents discussed the "best" places for training, they used for criteria the kinds of teaching, patients, and
responsibility they would have. For them the "best" internships
were those where they could learn the most medicine. Students
used these same criteria in choosing internships, but not in the
same way. A senior resident thus interpreted the remark quoted
above:

I would make a bet that Roget is just an outstanding student
who wanted to get a first-class internship in medicine, [and]
I think many people approach the internship like that, wanting
to get the best internship they can to learn the most they can.
[November 20, 1964]

Senior residents assume that students choose Boston City
Hospital because it is the "best" internship available. In fact,
students do choose what they consider to be the "best," but as
Roget explained, the "best" is a matter of reputation or prestige.
For students, "best" is not necessarily determined by the quality
of teaching, type of patient, or the interns' range of responsibility, though these are considered important. It is determined by
the reputation of the program and the medical setting.

Data gathered from the 1964 and 1965 interns at BCH indicates that two sets of criteria guided their choice of a program
and place at which to begin medical careers. Criteria for teaching, patients and responsibility were used when choosing "good"
internships—those that offered clinical experience that would
be a "good" base for whatever future career choices they might

make. Interns considered these particular criteria when judging a "good" clinical experience:

> "Well, I asked, "why did you choose BCH?" He said, "The thing I heard that I liked most about it was that you spent most of your time on the wards taking care of your own ward patients and that you didn't have to spend time on private wards taking care of patients for other doctors, as you do at a lot of other hospitals." He told me he had been at the Peter Bert Brigham as a student. I asked him if he had to take care of patients for doctors there, and he said, "Yes, I think there and Mass. General the intern doesn't have too much responsibility. It's just not so satisfactory a way to learn medicine as taking care of your own patients. You are not really taking responsibility of the patients. Here there are plenty of good people to advise you, if you want advice. But you are the patients' doctor." [June 18, 1965]

Students reported using teaching, patients, and responsibility as criteria in much the same way. Apparently they agree on what constitutes a "good" internship or clinical experience. Their use of these criteria does not differ from that of most other medical students. Everyone agrees that the internship should be a "good" clinical experience, characterized by a great deal of quality teaching, exposure to a variety of patients, and the opportunity to exercise medical responsibility.[14]

For students, however, "good" internships are not necessarily the "best." This latter category is related to, but not determined by, the quality of teaching, type of patients, or responsibility. Rather, it depends on the prestige of the program and its medical setting, as well as on the opportunity to make professional contacts. Students defined this last criterion as the opportunity to meet and work with established physicians, as well as to make friends who will be colleagues, moving in the same sphere of the medical world, at some time in the future. A sphere of medicine might be geographical or social, or might encompass a particular specialty or activity group. In either case, good professional contacts would facilitate travel along the career route.

14. For a discussion of criteria used by other students, see Becker and others, *Boys in White*, pp. 386–393.

A final criterion students used to judge their choice of internship was hospital facilities and working conditions. Interns at Boston City Hospital reported that they knew the facilities to be old and possibly inadequate. They also had considered the fact that there would be a heavy workload. "The working conditions," reported a medical student, "didn't influence my choice, but one can't ignore the dismal working conditions and facilities at the BCH." Another wrote, "One must ignore facilities and working conditions when applying to BCH." In fact, all students did ignore what they agreed were undesirable working conditions. The following comment illustrates the rationale for choosing an internship in terms of the two sets of criteria just discussed:

> I believe that there are, perhaps, 50 straight medical internships throughout the country that would provide as good training and experience; as good as any of those I applied to. The difference is one of prestige; important for anyone contemplating a career in academic medicine. [May 27, 1965]

THE DIRECTION AND DRIFT OF UNCOMMITTED CANDIDATES
FOR CAREERS

The choice of internships by students who did eventually come to Harvard resulted as much from an aversion to private practice as from any great affinity for the careers of academic medicine. Students chose those internships because the choice moved them along career routes away from private practice. They did not know exactly what the alternatives were, but they did know that alternatives would become available as they gained "good" clinical experience by serving one of the "best" internships of the medical profession. A university-affiliated internship, they know, does not preclude practice. It simply affords access to other routes as well.

A few students purposefully choose internships that advance their candidacies for elite careers. Most, however, simply attempted to increase the number of future careers that would be available to them. For them, the choice of an internship is influenced only slightly by elite aspirations. Attempting to avoid careers of medical practice, they choose internships that lend themselves to practice, research, or teaching, or a combination of these and by so choosing, place themselves on the route to the elite careers of medicine.

Many students who begin on the routes to elite medicine careers are only slightly aware of the kinds of careers open to them. If this is so, how can the interns at the Harvard Medical Unit be suitable candidates for the careers of academic medicine? Obviously, students whose aspirations do not encompass elite careers and who would be satisfied with general practice would not make suitable candidates. On the other hand, students attempting to advance their candidacies for elite careers and those who hope to avoid practice would use the same criteria when judging internships. Since both would be moving toward academic careers, they would make suitable, or at least potential, candidates for the careers of the medical elite.

Students moving away from practice are placed in positions from which they may drift into careers as scientists and teachers at schools of medicine. By choosing "name" internships, they become members of a pool of potential candidates who may be influenced to continue traveling toward the careers of the medical elite. As an intern on the Fourth (Harvard) Medical Service makes the point that efforts to find alternatives to practice often make students drift toward academic medicine:

> Alwin told me that Boston City Hospital wasn't his first choice, but that he was happy here and now jokes about his first choice, the Massachusetts General Hospital. He said, "We kind of kid a lot about the General. Most òf us feel that we are happy here. I had the General as my first choice. Others had The City as their first choice, probably could have gone either place. Comes down to six of one and a half-dozen of the other."
>
> I asked why he chose the General first and he replied, "The General is known all over the country, and their people go all over. Here, Thorndike has the reputation of turning out, you know, educators, and so on, but I think that may be a little . . . well, it's hard to say. It was certainly true in the past. You never quite know. Some people think the Thorndike

is dropping behind. I think the Medical Services are very good, but I honestly think that the fame of The City is due entirely to the Thorndike. But I think the Medical Services are good and they get good people to come here. All the people who become assistant professors come from the Thorndike."

I asked, "What about people from the Medical Services?"

Alwin nodded his head and said, "They do. A common pattern seems to be, since they are so strong in most clinical divisions of medicine, when you finish on the Medical Services you go on to the Thorndike. Then, from the Thorndike you stay or go elsewhere."

"What are your plans?" I asked Alwin.

He said, "Well, I'll get a fellowship in [a subspecialty] with [a 'name' physician]." I asked him if he planned to do this before he interned at Boston City Hospital.

"No. I was forced to make a decision because I didn't want to go down to NIH. I didn't care for the job that was available, so I stayed with the Berry Plan. That means I have to have a fellowship going into the assistant residency. The people going into the army or Public Health Service don't have to worry about it for a couple of years. I had to do some thinking and narrowed it down to a few specialities and then, suddenly, I decided it would be [that specialty]." He looked serious and said, "Not exactly. It did sort of creep up on me. Yes, it did. If I hadn't been in Part 2 of the Berry Plan and knew I would have to go into the army, I would have snapped at NIH. I might have gotten swept into some field that I started in down there."

I asked, "How would you get swept into a field of medicine?"

He replied, "If I did two years of work in a field, I probably would have discovered something interesting about it. There is nothing about the Cancer Institute that I particularly liked, but if I were to work there for two years maybe I would have become interested in it; a lot of people do. It does represent a substantial investment of time." [June 2, 1965]

At first I assumed that this intern planned an academic career and was illustrating the contingencies of travel along a route toward it. Later in our conversation, however, he indicated that he was drifting toward but was not yet entirely committed to a career of teaching and/or research.

I asked Alwin where else he would have liked to serve an internship. He told me that he had applied to Yale, Johns Hopkins, and a number of other well-known programs. "They are all famous," I said. He replied, "I think what people try to do when they decide that they are going into academic medicine is just get the best currency and training they can." "Currency?" I asked. Alwin nodded. "Yes, in terms of the best people. I feel that if you get the best training you are mobile, and you can go anywhere you want."

I asked, "Do you think you are able to trade in this currency you now have for a good fellowship and good academic employment?" Again he nodded, "I think that's probably true."

"Is that what you plan to do, go into academic medicine?"

"Well, I'm not sure yet. I'm not a big lab man, and I don't want that to be a major part of my life. I really would like to teach and would like to visit on the wards. Things like that, but not to spend most of my time in the lab. I like clinical medicine."

Many say they know what careers they want ultimately. They even give their aspirations a name—saying they plan a career in a particular specialty or, more specifically, announcing the name of a man with whom they wish to work.

Kaline stopped to talk for a minute: "I'm going to go upstairs. It's almost time for the conference, and I don't want to be late." Alwin asked "Why not?" Kaline: "Dr. Freinkel is presenting. It's diabetes consultation rounds, and that is what I want to go into, diabetes. I hope to someday work with Freinkel. That's why I don't want to be late." [July 3, 1965]

Aspirations, however, are frequently more varied and less specific than this man's. Not everyone knows, even by the time he is a senior resident, what he wants as a medical career. The following, more typical comment illustrates the variety of aspirations and the varying degree of commitment found in interns and residents at Boston City Hospital.

We went up to Medical 5, where the senior resident [Lawrence] was waiting with Seeler, the Chief of the Second Medical Service. Lawrence was sitting at the head of the table, with Seeler at his right. Williams, the assistant resident, was also there, doing lab work with Kaline, one of the new interns.

We sat down, I asked Lawrence what he hoped to accomplish by holding the meeting. He answered that he thought it best to have things clear from the beginning, things about running the ward. I asked Lawrence what he planned to do after his residency at Boston City Hospital. He replied, "I'm from Ohio, and I think I would like to practice medicine in a small town." I asked the same question of Schwartz, who sat between Lawrence and me. He replied. "I plan to go into academic medicine. I always have. I guess that's why I'm here." He chuckled.

MacDougal, on my left, shook his head. When I asked him what was the matter, he said, "Well, everyone seems to be so sure of what they want to do. I know I'm interested in this new idea of electronic data processing, but that's all I know."

Kaline was sitting away from the table listening and, in an attempt to include him, Lawrence asked what his plans were. He said, "I plan on going into opthalmology." Lawrence nodded and said that was getting to be the thing. Williams asked, "Isn't anybody interested in what I'm going to do?" I laughed and said I was interested. He said, "You know what I'm gonna do? I'm gonna go into academic medicine." I laughed and said: "That's not very original." Everyone laughed. [June 29, 1965]

A lack of commitment to any particular career facilitates drift. The drifter travels career routes without a commitment to a particular career that would preclude travel along some routes of the medical profession. Consider, for example, the medical school graduate who accepts an internship in pathology. He may be advancing his candidacy for an academic career further than the students who choose to serve internships in medicine, but he is also making an early commitment that could rule out other medical careers. The same could be said of medical students who choose to serve no internship but do graduate work. Both of these students exhibit maximum commitment to particular careers. The drifter, on the other hand, is the least committed of candidates. He is looking for an internship that closes the door on no career and maximizes the number open to him. He tries to stay uncommitted for as long as possible.[15]

Some elite careers could grow out of a series of defaulting

15. The characteristics of a drifter are discussed by David Matza, *Delinquency and Drift* (New York, John Wiley, 1964).

decisions and not elite aspirations or prudent choice and action. In this chapter I have attempted to describe the first default that initiates the movement toward the elite medical careers. Possibly there are other defaults. Further progress along these career routes may be similar, and other critical choices may be made accidentally. The interns were, in fact, making just this sort of progress toward careers in medicine. Most were drifters.[16]

The recruitment of drifters as interns is an excellent way to staff the Harvard Medical Service. Since he is uncommitted, the drifter does not have an interest in obtaining one and only one kind of training. The experience of caring for patients is sufficient for whatever subsequent career moves he will make, as long as the internship he serves "looks good on paper." This means that there is no inherent conflict between what interns are expected to do and what they want or are willing to do. Interns who are drifters are willing to spend their time attending patients to obtain credentials which will permit them to progress further toward desirable careers. That is, since they are uncommitted they are more likely to accept a definition of their training which facilitates the purpose of the Harvard Medical Unit.

All young men who are committed are also potential candidates for other positions at the Harvard Medical Unit. They will, for example, be available to fill the positions of assistant residents. During the year they could also develop a commitment which would be both cause and effect of elite aspirations. That is, these young men could acquire elite aspirations and become committed to those careers after they actually begin on a route to elite medical careers. Since this is likely to occur, by choosing drifters the Harvard Medical Unit assures itself of sufficient candidates for the careers it advocates in medicine. And, if this does not occur, at least these young men are willing to do the work of an internship.

16. A few of the interns I observed in 1965 were drifting as late as 1968, when they made application for fellowships at the Center for Community Health and Medical Care. At no time did interns discuss the possibility of careers in community health, but four years later, some were in search of those careers. They had somehow made their way to the first positions on the ladder of a relatively new career in medicine.

The uncommitted candidate for a professional career has received little attention, but the drifter may be more characteristic of professional trainees than is usually assumed. A sociological model that makes no allowance for the ways people drift into careers explains the course of travel of only some candidates for the profession. My study of Harvard interns suggests a model for professional training that would include uncommitted candidates and defaulting decisions. Such a model may prove useful in explaining the decision-making processes that affect travel along the routes of other professions. Sociologically, the beginnings of those careers were the result of efforts by recruiters to assure themselves of suitable candidates for the careers they were advocating and of decisions by students that intentionally placed them on routes taking them away from a traditional medical career but accidentally made them candidates for the careers of the medical elite.[17]

17. For example, Delbert Miller and W. H. Form, *Industrial Sociology* (New York, Harper, 1957). I am aware of the criticism of a position emphasizing occupational choices as accidents by such people as Ginzberg and others. *Occupational Choice* (New York, Columbia University Press, 1951). There is only slightly more evidence, in my opinion, for considering occupational choice rational than there is for a position emphasizing the choice of direction but postulating a principle of double-effect such as I have described.

5. The Work of an Internship

ONCE AN internship that provides satisfactory credentials without requiring an irrevocable commitment has been obtained, an intern's future aspirations become less important than the immediate job of successfully completing the work of an internship. The work consists almost entirely of attending patients in emergency rooms, clinics, and on the wards. Some interns begin by admitting and caring for patients on the wards. Others start out in the clinics or on the accident floor. A few have no patients of their own at first, but supplement the efforts of interns on the wards by assisting them in the evening and caring for their patients at night. At any time during the year, most of the interns are working on the wards, while the others are assigned duties off the wards.

An internship is supposed to be an educational experience which prepares men for the practice of medicine. When they arrive at the hospital, interns anticipate having a great deal to do, and are willing to do it because they believe it will make them better physicians. They do, of course, gain experience by taking medical histories, doing physical examinations, and making diagnoses, but the bulk of what they do is not pertinent to what their work will be in the future. The work certainly is not like that of the academic physicians they see at the hospital. Much of their work is not even like that of practicing physicians. A physician in private practice, for example, does not do routine laboratory tests, nor does he have to run around the hospital to supplement his treatment plans for patients. Their work in clinics, a setting most like the "doctor's office," also differs from the practice they are likely to have because the patients they see are not typical of those who consult private physicians. The internship, therefore, is not so much an educational experience approximating the work of full-fledged physicians as it is a particular kind of job at Boston City Hospital.

By doing his job, the work assigned to him, the intern contributes to the hospital's program of patient care. Technically, interns are employees of the hospital. They must carry out the duties delegated and regulated by administrators and physicians who have their own purposes, only incidentally related to training physicians. Thus the purpose of an intern's work is dictated by the objectives of the hospital and the purposes of the physicians responsible for his training. If the objectives of the hospital and purposes of the physicians staffing it are to be advanced, the purpose of an intern's work must be the provision of patient care. That is what interns are expected to do and it is what they actually do during the year.

Simply, the hospital needs interns to meet the demand for medical care, to discharge its obligation to the public. The work could be done by graduates of any medical school, but the graduates of any school would not also serve the purposes of the Harvard Medical Unit.

The work that an intern must do is explained in memoranda describing ward and clinic assignments and the duties entailed, and further stipulated by the conditions of his employment by the hospital. Interns learn in this way and are also told by other people what is formally required of them as employees of Boston City Hospital. What is described in this chapter is the required work of an internship. Though the work is required, it may or may not provide the particular experiences that interns are searching for by serving an internship.

What is formally required of an intern best serves the purposes of Boston City Hospital and the Harvard Medical Unit. The required work of an internship may not, however, provide the educational experiences sought by medical school graduates. Though I discuss the processes by which interns learn to do what is required of them and the tactics they employ to accomplish their own purposes in subsequent chapters, I will indicate in this chapter what the differences are between the purposes of serving an internship and the purpose of work that interns must do as employees of the Boston City Hospital.

THE WORK ON THE WARDS

There is a maxim that concisely defines the responsibility of an intern and his relationship to other house officers: "The patient belongs to the intern; the ward belongs to the assistant resident; a medical service belongs to the senior resident; and both services belong to the chief resident." The intern has been told since his student days that responsibility for the patient is the hallmark of the physician. The opportunity to exercise responsibility is attractive to an intern because it is a benchmark of his progress in medicine and because it enables him to deal directly with patients and thereby gain valued clinical experience.

Clinical experience comes from learning by doing; it consists of knowledge about disease and exposure to actual medical problems, the base of any medical career. Interns look forward eagerly to the almost seven months of the year they will spend on the male and female wards. As a member of a group consisting of another intern or two, the assistant resident, medical students, and nurses, the intern will divide his time almost equally between the two wards. Other physicians are assigned as visiting staff on a rotating basis. These visiting physicians act primarily as teachers and take little part in caring for patients.

An intern's day on the ward begins between seven and eight

The Work of an Internship : 93

in the morning. He arrives early to meet with the assistant resident, take the report of the "night float," the intern who relieved him the previous evening and may have admitted new patients, or attend to laboratory work. All these things are done before he makes his rounds, which he does from about eight until ten every day but Sunday, usually accompanied by the assistant resident and medical students. This team sees each patient and discusses his medical problems as well as the plan for his medical care. The intern presents the patients assigned to him and explains what he plans to do for them and why. These activities are not work rounds in the sense that work is actually done, though on occasion a procedure may be performed or something that has been decided at the moment may be done there and then. If, for example, it is decided that a patient would benefit from sitting up, a chair may be brought and the patient assisted out of bed. This is not, however, the purpose of work rounds. Most of the time is spent presenting new patients or discussing the problems and treatment of old patients.

When the intern and the assistant resident both know the patients and agree on treatment plans, work rounds progress quickly. It is at this time that decisions are made. When patients are presented, other staff, particularly the assistant resident, will comment on the diagnosis and plans made by the intern. At this time the intern informs other interns, students, and the assistant resident of the results of the physical examination and the group either agrees with the diagnosis and treatment plan or offers alternatives. The following are typical examples of what happens during work rounds.

> The house staff was having difficulty in agreeing on the diagnosis and deciding on a plan of treatment. Marrio, the assistant resident, asked, "What about steroids?" Lowenthal, the intern, shakes his head and says, "I don't think we have a clean diagnosis. It might be cirrhosis. I don't think steroids are indicated." Marrio agrees that is a good point; Lowenthal suggests doing a biopsy. A medical student and the senior resident agree with Lowenthal who turns to Marrio and asks, "Do you think I'm wrong? If you do, I'll send him home today." Marrio

shakes his head and says, "No, I think you can ask for a biopsy." Lowenthal nods and makes a note in the patient chart. [July 17, 1964]

At other times, the diagnosis is clear but there is some question about the treatment:

The patient had a myocardial infarct. An assistant resident said: "We keep them in bed for three weeks. Up in a chair the early part of the fourth week. Discharge is about the fifth week." Smith, an intern, looked surprised and said, "No kidding. Really?" The assistant resident told him that was the treatment for a myocardial infarction. Smith asked, "What do you think of that?"

"Obviously," replied the assistant resident, "if we are doing it here on the ward, I like it. What do you think?"

Smith: "It's so different from what I'm used to. We usually [as a medical student at another hospital] had them up in 36 hours. Do you have any trouble with phlebitis?"

The assistant resident nodded and said, "We have had some, but you just have to watch for it. We could do it your way [but] we haven't the equipment. If we did, your way would be better. Here, this way is best." The intern makes a note on some cards he is carrying. We moved on to the next patient. [July 27, 1965]

The purpose of work rounds is explained by interns thus:

I asked, "What is the good of work rounds?" "Well, for one thing," answered the intern, "it's good for the patient, because you are discussing that patient's care. You want to find out what's wrong with him. Work rounds aren't for discussion of all the physiology of what's going on. Of course, you do. But work rounds are just to find out what's happening to the patient. That's the time to check things out, sort of everyday things. What you want to talk about is what's going on and what should be done for this particular patient." [May 25, 1965]

Work rounds end at ten. At that time, the assistant resident leaves the ward to attend a meeting with other residents, where he reports the condition and disposition of patients on his ward. While the assistant resident is away and before conferences or visiting rounds, which begin at 10:30, interns are free. During this half-hour they may do some of the things that were recommended during work ·rounds or write orders and requests for things they want other hospital personnel to do for their patients. They may take a coffee break, but even coffee time is related to their work. The morning coffee break is one of the few times they have to sit during their work day. A break in the routine, as the following incident illustrates, is important.

> A new intern on the ward, Benson, and I entered the kitchen, off the ward. He sat down and started to write in the black book for doctor's orders. Koren, who has been on the ward for a month or so, walks in and says, "I agree, I think it's best to sit down and write your orders. It's too hard to write while moving along [on work rounds]." Benson says, "I always make mistakes when I write as we're walking." Although he had been told by the assistant resident to write his orders immediately after seeing the patient, he waited until he could sit down and do so over a cup of coffee. Koren got a cup of coffee for himself and waited for the order book. [July 31, 1964]

The half-hour between 10 and 10:30 is the only "free" time that interns have during the morning. On Monday, Wednesday, and Friday from 10:30 to noon they make visiting rounds on the wards. On other days the latter part of the morning is reserved for special conferences or consultation rounds with staff members of the research divisions and affiliated clinics. "In the middle of the morning," explained an intern, "it's convenient to have a half-hour to use to do chores and catch up on your work."

Interns break for lunch at noon, though their lunch may be interrupted by lectures or conferences. These conferences may be a presentation of an interesting patient by a medical student, or the more formal conferences involving physicians from one or all three of the medical schools at the hospitals. If interns attend these conferences, and they usually do, they have time for nothing more than a quick lunch before going to the clinic or returning to the wards.

On the wards, interns do much the same kinds of things during the afternoon. One of them, for example, is "on call." When he is on call he is the admitting intern and receives all new patients admitted to his ward during the day. The patients he admits are permanently assigned to him, and he assumes responsibility for their care.

The admitting intern devotes his afternoon to working up new patients. Working up patients consists of taking medical histories, doing physical examinations, and making diagnoses. In addition, the intern must do routine laboratory tests. He may draw a blood sample or get a urine or stool specimen which he will examine later. There is a laboratory on or near the ward where he may do blood counts, urinalyses, and other routine tests. Most afternoons are spent in the laboratory or on the wards performing diagnostic and therapeutic procedures.

After writing up his patients, an intern writes up his findings, entering all pertinent information in each patient's chart. As soon as possible after admission, the assistant resident in charge of the ward also examines each patient and writes a "note," a summary of his opinion of the diagnostic and therapeutic problems of each patient. Though the patient "belongs" to the intern, the assistant resident has the authority to decide the treatment he will receive. Interns must review every case with the assistant resident. Together they appraise each patient's condition and evaluate the intern's plan of treatment. If the intern's work-up has not yielded sufficient information for an objective appraisal, he may have to return to the patient for additional information or request special diagnostic tests. When interns are not on call, they use most of their time to bring charts up-to-date, discuss patients with the assistant resident, and arrange to obtain any additional information and assistance they may need to make diagnoses and facilitate treatment plans.

Though it may later be revised, a plan of care for each patient is implemented almost immediately. Interns begin to do things for a patient as soon as they have some idea of his condition and problems. They spend more time, however, in working up patients and arranging for consultation and special diagnostic tests than in performing therapeutic procedures.

Working up new patients and caring for those already admitted is only part of an intern's work. He must also see that his requests are met and his related orders carried out by other hospital personnel. Requesting X-rays, for example, is only the beginning of all that he must do to get a film he can use. Many times porters are not available to transport patients, so interns may have to take them to the laboratory. After the X-rays are taken, interns may still have to keep after technicians to process the film; once they are ready, the intern may call for the films himself, rather than wait for them to be delivered to the ward. Another example is the patient's chart. If the patient has previously been at the hospital, there is a chart containing his medical history and past problems. Since the intern needs that information almost immediately, he must make frequent trips to the hospital's medical records department. All in all, a large part of each afternoon consists of "running around" the hospital. Many interns report spending as much time running around the hospital as they do with their patients. The following comment is typical.

> On our way back to the ward from X-ray, Woolcot said, "This is how I spend much of my time. We have to run around and make sure things get done. The nurse may say the X-ray was sent over and that it's there, but you have to run it down. At some other hospitals, maybe, you just write a ticket and things get done. Here, you have to make sure. Sometimes, you have to do them yourself." [June 10, 1964]

Later in the afternoon, before or after supper, the interns and the assistant resident again make rounds. The intern on call spends the night at the hospital. During these rounds, those who are not on call inform the one who is and the assistant resident of any problems they anticipate. All interns more or less turn over their patients during the evening to the intern on duty, who cares for them until late in the evening. In fact, the turning over of responsibility is largely symbolic. An intern must remain at the hospital until he has completed his work. "At no time," interns are told, "shall the intern leave without completing his work, recording it, and informing the intern on call of the ward problems."

For the intern the early evening hours are not much different from the afternoon. Most hospital departments have closed for the day so there is less "running around." But the intern continues to draw blood, collect specimens, do routine laboratory tests, bring patient's charts up-to-date, write requests and orders, and perform therapeutic procedures. It is to his advantage to do as much as he can that day, because the next day he may be on call, seeing new patients and having other work to do. Most interns work late into the evening, remaining at the hospital until the "night float" reports for duty.

One intern on each service acts as night float, coming on duty shortly after ten in the evening. The float does not replace the intern on call, who must remain at the hospital. After 10:30 P.M. admitting and working up new patients is the responsibility of the night float. If he cannot handle all the work, he may request the intern on call to help with admissions or to treat patients. In the morning the night float presents each new patient admitted, as well as any significant changes in the condition of others. With his report, another day of work begins.

There is no doubt that "running around" facilitates the delivery of patient care, which is the purpose of the hospital. There is little if anything interns do when running around, however, that adds significantly to their clinical experience or knowledge of medicine. The same can be said of the time that interns spend doing routine laboratory tests on specimens that they themselves had to obtain from patients. The running around and laboratory work that interns do is nothing more than what they must do as employees of Boston City Hospital.

THE WORK OFF THE WARDS

Like most hospitals, Boston City Hospital provides emergency services and operates an outpatient department. One of the busiest of these facilities is the accident floor, to which people come or are brought in off the streets. Equally familiar are the clinics: open clinics, at which people who think themselves in need of general medical attention are screened, attended to, or routed elsewhere for further attention; appointment clinics, for patients who return to a specific physician; and the specialty clinics, which provide a particular sort of medical attention. Interns are required to participate in all these activities, except the specialty clinics, and are off the wards for approximately two and a half months seeing patients on the accident floor or at outpatient clinics.

Each month one intern is assigned the accident floor with a resident, while others are scheduled to attend to patients at the open medical clinic. Those in the outpatient department arrange a float schedule, which allows one of them to assist at the afternoon clinic. Monday through Friday, beginning at 8:30 A.M., interns at the open clinic see patients, either those new to the hospital or those who have not attended the clinic for a year. Clinic patients who come to the hospital without appointments are assigned to an intern. The purpose of the clinic is explained by the following comments of an assistant resident:

> I think the clinic here is sort of . . . well, the morning clinic at any rate, is sort of a necessary evil in that there is a big population in Boston that has got to be seen by somebody. It's sort of like the accident floor. It's dumping ground, so to speak, in that you see a lot of trivial stuff but, once again, I think this can be a valuable thing in that this is the way medicine is. You've got to know how to approach a patient with a head injury or a guy with a lacerated hand, as well as knowing how to manage a guy with a heart attack. The clinic is a little bit different from the accident floor. You get things like headaches and sore throats and fainting spells and things like that; you see a lot of insignificant problems. Yet, you do serve a very useful function out there because you do see people who don't have any doctor and they come and they do have a complaint and you're their first and last line of defense. You go out there and you see these people and you have to make decisions on them. Do they really have a genuine complaint? What is your plan going to be? You have to decide if they can be handled on the outside or if they need hospitalization . . . you become their doctor. [December 15, 1964]

Many people in Boston who do not have a regular physician think of the medical clinic at Boston City Hospital as the place to go when they want medical care. Needless to say, not all of them are sick, and a good number of those who are need only some immediate remedy. People who come to the morning clinic confront house officers with random encounters for which they are not completely prepared and about which they must obtain information before determining proper medical approach.[1] Of course, interns perform a variety of trivial medical procedures, but most of their activity consists of working up patients about whom they know little. The patient charts are a reliable source of information about people who have been at the hospital before, but these are not always available. For first-time visitors, no charts are available. Chart or no, the intern asks the patient about his symptoms and performs a physical examination, seeking signals that will tell him how sick the patient is and what action is warranted. He attends to those who need immediate treatment and evolves plans for handling those who are sick enough to require further outpatient care or admission to the hospital. His decisions depend on obtaining information and, as the following comments indicate, he is given a great deal of independence:

> Schlereth, who had been night float but now was at OPD [outpatient department], joined us for lunch. Doyle asked him how he liked OPD. Schlereth said, "It's a ball! You get to make all sorts of definitive decisions. Do this! Don't do that! I hear the accident floor is even better." [July 28, 1964]

> On the way over from clinic to Peabody 3 [the building housing the Fourth Medical Service], I asked Blocksberg what he thought he did most of during clinic. He said, "Getting information from the patient. I think that's the major thing we do on the ward too, or should be doing on the ward. This is more obvious in clinic. We also are much more on our own, make our own decisions." [September 10, 1964]

1. Interns at morning clinic face social situations similar to those of a salesman facing customers who have simply "dropped in" at a retail store. Since he is not completely prepared for this "cold call," the salesman often finds it difficult to determine a proper sales approach. An intern likewise attempts to evolve hypotheses about this particular patient and modify his action in terms of his understanding. Cf. Stephen J. Miller, "The Social Base of Sales Behavior," *Social Problems*, 12, 1 (Summer, 1964), pp. 15–24.

The intern's participation in the outpatient department is not limited to the morning medical clinic. One day a week he is assigned to the outpatient building, where interns staff the afternoon medical clinic. Unlike the morning clinic, this one is not "open," but is specifically reserved for patients receiving continuing medical care and for those referred from morning cinics. Most afternoon patients have recently required hospitalization. Either they have been the intern's patients on the ward, or he has inherited them during a formal exchange of clinic patients held at the beginning of the year.

Through this exchange, patients of departing house officers are allotted to incoming interns. Together with those he himself admits to clinic from the wards, they become his continuing responsibility throughout his stay at the hospital.

Though the hospital tries to regulate the number of people coming to the clinic by giving afternoon patients appointments with specific house officers, still some drop by to see the doctor. This, however, is not so much a problem for the intern as it is in the morning. Since these people have been at clinic before, information about them is available. If he has the patient's chart, he need not do a complete physical or conduct an extensive inquiry; he knows the medical histories. Not everyone comes to the clinic with a documented past, but interns come to know their patients well.

> I have learned the lesson of following your patients carefully so you can anticipate problems . . . you're right on your patients. I really found this to be valuable in the clinic. I have a whole raft of people there whom I really got to know, who are my friends, and when something is wrong I really know. I have a woman in the clinic who never had a complaint for four months, as long as I have known her. Suddenly, she had a severe headache. I admitted her to the hospital right away, and she had blood in her head. [May 19, 1965]

An intern himself sometimes admits to the afternoon clinic people who have been his patients on the wards. He has already worked them up, prescribed for them and treated them while they were in the hospital. Another examination and further interrogation would add little to the knowledge he already has. He is their doctor.

> You nurse them through their period of sickness and then you become their doctor, from then until the time you leave. You set up your appointments. You have your afternoon out there. You've got your own office, your own examining table, and your own desk. Nobody supervises you. You know, nobody sitting out there saying, "OK, you listen to the heart or lung." You do what you want to and follow up on those patients. This is the way office practices would be. The burden of good medical practice falls on you, because here you don't have the assistant resident or the senior resident, anybody, looking over your shoulder, watching how you manage your clinic patients. If you got a guy with a bad lung or heart and he comes in and you don't listen to his lungs or heart, well, there's nobody there to say that you've got to listen to his lungs or you'd better listen to his heart or you've got to take his blood pressure or you'd better feel his pulse. You're a grown-up doctor. [December 15, 1964]

Not all interns are happy about the demands made on them by their duties at the outpatient department. Opinion regarding the clinic experience ranges from a succinct "It's a pain in the ass," to an enthusiastic "It's a great experience." Interns' statements repeatedly stress that participation in the activity of the outpatient, particularly the morning, clinic is necessary but not too important for their training. Work at the clinics is something that simply must be done.

> "The clinic, I think, is a good experience when you follow the patients that you have had on the ward, but I think it's unsatisfactory when you are seeing new patients. No privacy, and you see a lot of them in a short time. It goes very quickly."
>
> I asked, "You prefer following your own patients to getting new ones in the A.M. clinic?"
>
> Rod replied, "I think you learn more if you follow your own patients. The benefit of a clinic, as far as I'm concerned, is a chance to follow the course of the patients over a long time, to see how they do. The formal purpose of a clinic is to keep them going, take care of them there without admitting

them to the hospital. Also, a lot has to do with welfare, evaluating patients for various kinds of disabilities. This is a valid purpose for the community. So in the clinic I think you are performing a useful role, but I don't think you are learning a lot by doing it unless [the person] turns out to be a patient you will follow over a long period of time. [June 18, 1965]

Patients at the morning clinic require a lengthy initial examination, but usually there is no reason for continuing medical care. Most of the effort consists of providing immediate but minor medical attention. Similarly, interns consider the accident floor to be a part of their job that must be done rather than an opportunity to follow patients:

> I said to Andy, "Over on emergency, it looks like it's more slap-and-patch than anything else." He replied, "Well, that's why I say the major thing you can hope to achieve there, at least in this hospital, is to decide if a person is sick enough to be admitted. If they need only ambulatory care you refer them to the outpatient department or the appropriate physician on the accident floor. I don't think you are, by any stretch of the imagination, able to give care on the accident floor. There are too many patients for the number of doctors, and that's why in many respects all you are accomplishing there, at least for a large number of patients, is just routing them to where they can get proper care." [May 3, 1965]

On the accident floor the intern encounters situations that require decisions based on little medical information. No matter what the complaint, the intern must see each patient, sometimes as many as 150 in an eight-hour day. He provides immediate care to those who need nothing more, and admits to the hospital those who need more extensive attention. The sheer number of patients he must see prohibits him from doing more than examining for a diagnosis. In short, his examination is geared to decide if the patient is sick enough to be admitted to the hospital. The patients he admits will probably not become his. "You can follow patients that you've admitted to see what happens to them, but it's not often done." [2] The intern will see

2. *Intern,* June 18, 1965.

afternoon clinic patients over a period of time. He will have an opportunity to watch the course of an illness or observe his patients' progress outside the hospital. This chance for follow-up constitutes what the interns consider the most valuable part of their experience off the wards. (See Table 5.1).

Table 5.1. Types of Statements Made by Interns to Describe Clinic Experience at Boston City Hospital, 1964, 1965

Content of statement	Type of clinic	Number of statements
"It's a service."	A.M.	9
	P.M.	3
"It's very much like a small practice of your own. You get to make all kinds of definitive decisions."	A.M. and P.M.	18
"It's a good way to follow your patients."	A.M.	0
	P.M.	11
Total		41

Another aspect of the clinic work is its similarity to a medical practice. One afternoon a week interns are able to prescribe for patients and, at some later date, evaluate any change they may have effected. Much of what interns do, of course, is like the activity of a practice, but the coming and going of patients they may never see again and the kinds of patients they do see are hardly representative of a typical practice. Thus interns make the comparison with reservations, noting discrepancies between their outpatient experiences and a medical practice:

> I asked if clinic was like a medical practice. Scott said, "In a way, but not exactly." I asked how it was different, and he replied, "For one, the way these people live. Practices are mostly with middle class patients, and these aren't middle class patients."
> I asked, "What does that mean?" Scott: "Well, you have to

take this into account when you ask them to do something. They may not do it. You can bet that they're not going to do a lot of the things they should or you want them to do. The middle class patient will, I think."

I asked, "Then why the clinic for the intern?" Scott: "I think it provides services for the community. It's something the hospital has to do." [September 21, 1964]

Clearly, the patients that come to the outpatient department are not typical of the patients who consult private physicians. They reflect a level of health below that of most middle-income groups in America. Interns are quick to point out that a major characteristic of the clinic patient population is its lack of information about "proper" health practices and habits.

Mayer told me about his next patient: "She's a 15-year-old who's just started having sexual relations and has a urinary tract infection." The girl entered the examining room and Mayer said, "Hello, Jane. Why don't you sit down? How have you been feeling?" The girl closed her eyes, shrugged her shoulders, and nodded her head. Mayer asked: "Have you and your boyfriend been taking any precautions?" When the girl looked at him as if she didn't understand, he explained: "Have you been using anything?" The girl shook her head. Mayer: "What would happen if you got pregnant?" The girl shrugged her shoulders. "Are you trying to get pregnant?" The girl shook her head. Mayer nodded and said: "Why don't you get into that dressing gown? We'll be back in a minute."

We stepped outside, but didn't go anywhere. Mayer said, "The problem is that they have no concept of basic hygiene. They really complicate their lives at such an early age. This girl doesn't even know how to douche."

He turned and we entered the examining room, where the girl was sitting up on the examining table. I sat down on a chair and Mayer examined the girl. When he finished, he wrote a prescription and said, "Now, Jane, I want you to take these now. It's important that you take them as soon as possible. I think they'll cost about $6. Do you have $6?" The girl said her mother gave her only $5.

"Will you be able to get the money today?" "No, not until tomorrow. My mother is out." "Then I want you to get as many as $5 will get you. You should start taking these right away. It's important. You're a young girl now, and if you take care of this, you'll have no trouble, but if you let it go, then you'll have a lot of trouble when you get to be a lady." He then explained the procedure for taking the medicine and asked the girl to repeat it. [September 10, 1964]

Interns consider it important to be able to observe how people fare after they are discharged from the hospital. The afternoon clinic gives them this experience of caring for people throughout the course of a variety of illnesses. Further, clinics afford an opportunity to exercise medical responsibility. Being required to diagnose and determine the disposition of people who come to the clinic and the making of definitive decisions makes work off the wards worthwhile. The exercise of responsibility is, however, considered to be less valuable than the experience of following patients during the posthospital phase of illness. When the circumstances of work do not permit follow-up on patients, interns consider what they do to be a legitimate but unrewarding activity.

ACADEMIC ACTIVITY

Along with their on-the-job training, interns attend formal lectures and conferences as well as such less formal teaching sessions as the "visiting rounds." The most familiar tableau of medical education is the grouping of students, interns, and teaching physicians around the bed of a patient, all listening to an old and wise physician. Actually, interns spend no more than 10 per cent of their time making rounds with visiting teaching physicians.

Visiting rounds take place three or four days a week, between 10:30 and noon. The format and content are determined by the interests of the visiting physicians (see Chapter 6). They may be conducted as a seminar held away from the wards or in the more traditional round of patients on the wards. Visiting physicians who teach in the sequence of training interns are usually staff members of a research division at the Thorndike Memorial Laboratory. Occasionally, however, they may be young specialists practicing in Boston and seeking an affiliation with the Harvard Medical Unit.

The more academically oriented of the physicians who conduct visiting rounds prefer the seminar format, like that described below, which was conducted by a member of a research division involved in clinical and laboratory studies.

We entered the laboratory on the third floor of Peabody, where we were to meet Dr. Flener, the visiting physician. Dr. Flener and the assistant resident were sitting with their backs to the door, facing the group of students and interns. Schwartz, a student, began the discussion by presenting a patient case: a white 74-year-old male with G.I. bleeding. When he finished, Flener asked, "What about the test results?" Schwartz asked if he wanted all the results, and Flener shook his head. "No, just give me the important ones; those that showed something, or those that didn't show something but, for that reason, are important." Schwartz gave the results of blood tests and urinanalysis, and described a mass he felt in the abdomen.

Flener asked if anyone else had felt the mass, and Smith, an intern, said he had. Flener wanted to know if Schwartz had described the mass accurately. Smith said, "I think it was larger than that, probably 4 to 5 rather than 2 to 4 inches." Schwartz then volunteered the information that the patient denied that he drank a great deal, but that he and Smith did not believe the patient. Flener asked Schwartz to describe the mass in detail and after he did, wanted a diagnosis. Schwartz said he thought it was an ulcer.

Flener asked what Schwartz would do about the ulcer, saying, "Here we have a really good one for a medical-surgical give and take. The patient is 74 years old and can't stand too much surgery. We could medicate him, but he may bleed again. There are pros and cons on both sides." Schwartz responded that he would recommended surgery. Smith and the others agreed, Smith saying, "I thing that statistics show that in 76 per cent of the cases where medical management of ulcers was attempted, patients had surgery anyway. I don't think we will be able to manage the ulcer, and we might as well have the surgery done now." There then was a very technical discussion of what kind of surgery, a partial resectioning or a full resectioning. Flener said, quite emphatically:

"A man of 74 won't stand a complete surgical job. I'd just suggest a partial resectioning." That ended the discusson of that patient.

Bloomfield, the assistant resident, told Flener that there was one other patient to be presented before we visited the wards. Smith presented the second patient: a 50-year-old male admitted to the hospital for the first time with no past history of cirrhosis and denying that he drank heavily or had lost weight. Smith gave the results of all the tests he ran and concluded it was a case of cirrhosis complicated by diabetes. Bloomfield said, "Well, we seem to be agreed on that, but what if we accept the patient at his word? He says he's not a heavy drinker; let's assume he's not." Smith shook his head and said he was certain the patient was a heavy drinker. Bloomfield said, "I'm just trying to make this interesting." Looking at Smith, he again added: "What if we do accept the man's word?" Someone said, "Hemochromatosis" [a disease of the skin and viscera affecting pigmentation, called "bronzed diabetes"]. Flener laughed and asked, "Do you really want me to get started on that?" He then described the drinking habits of an African tribe frequently suffering from cirrhosis and hemochromatosis. Flener reviewed relevant publications, beginning with a monograph published in 1935, and went on to explain the social and biological conditions thought to account for the disease. His concluding remark was that there was not enough data and that the topic would be an interesting one to study.

Although he talked about this for a good half-hour, everyone agreed that the original diagnosis was correct. I had the feeling that Smith and Bloomfield had purposely led the discussion to a topic that was of interest to Flener. Only 3 per cent of the Africans drinking iron-loaded beer suffer from hemochromatosis, so it's unlikely that the disease is a big problem at Boston City Hospital. By the time Flener finished, we were behind schedule. Bloomfield led the group out of the lab and to the ward where they made an abbreviated round of patients. [June 10, 1964]

In contrast to an academic discussion of interesting diseases are the patient-by-patient rounds, usually conducted by physicians interested in patient care as well as the study of the disease.

Peterson, Hink, Schwartz, and I left the laboratory on Peabody 3 to return to the ward and meet Dr. Blocksberg, a clinical associate, who was the visiting physician for June. Freeman, the assistant resident, introduced us to Dr. Blocksberg. As we entered the ward, Blocksberg said, "I think we will just look around at the patients and see what you have." The first patient was a white female with an ulceration, presented to Blocksberg by the intern Hink. Dr. Blocksberg was concerned that the students and I (at the back of the group) were not hearing the presentation and repeatedly asked Hink to speak up. The next patient was presented by Peterson, who was immediately told to speak up. This patient was a female admitted for a myocardial infarct; she had been in bed for ten days.

After examining her, Blocksberg asked Peterson what he was doing for her. Peterson told him what medication he had prescribed. Blocksberg said, "That's good. That's standard procedure. How about getting her up out of bed? Can't we tie her comfortably in a chair?" Before Peterson could answer, Freeman asked, "Sir, don't you agree with our policy here of complete bedrest for an MI?" Blocksberg said it could be done both ways, explaining: "I think that older people deteriorate very rapidly in bed. That it's better to get them up in a chair. They have by this age developed some collateral circulation. The younger patient who hasn't developed any degree of collateral circulation would be treated differently." Peterson was nodding his head. Freeman said, "I would tend to agree with you that the patients when they are older deteriorate in bed, but (pointing to a chair) you can see that we don't have the best equipment. I know that over at the Brigham they have special chairs, but here we just have these straight wooden chairs." Blocksberg said the equipment was not the best, but that something could be worked out. Then he told us of how he treats a 96-year-old female: "I have never had her on complete bedrest, and she's had infarcts twice."

We moved on to the next patient. The next patient, presented by Hink, was a middle-aged female who had been in the hospital for three days, running a fever of unknown origin. Blocksberg asked Hink what he thought, but Hink just shrugged his shoulders. Blocksberg asked what was being done for her, and Hink told him he had put her on sulfanilamide and asked what he would suggest. Blocksberg: "Well, before the days of wonder drugs and antibiotics we used ice-cold boric acid compresses, as cold as you can get them. Put the boric acid right in a bowl of ice cubes." Hink asked, "Four per cent solution?" Blocksberg laughed and said, "You can't do better than 4 per cent no matter how hard you try. Four per cent is it. Just put enough in so there's a little residual at the bottom that will be absorbed when the ice cubes melt."

The next patient was a jaundiced middle-aged female. Blocksberg examined the patient, palpating the liver. He said, "There is an unusual liver edge. If they haven't already felt this, the students should feel this. It's always good to feel a liver edge once." After his examination of the patient, he said, "I don't know too much about the liver, but I would certainly be interested in hearing the opinion of someone who does." A senior resident asked a few questions, but we had to go to a student conference, so this had to be the last patient for the day. [July 1, 1964]

Interns, students, and residents on a ward meet with the same visiting physician three or four mornings a week for a month. The purpose of visiting rounds is to inform interns, students, and residents about diseases and their management by bringing them together with physicians who have a great deal of specialized knowledge and experience in a particular area. The following comments illustrate why interns think specialists make good visiting physicians.

> With a visiting physician who specializes, you have the opportunity to discuss interesting cases in detail and go into a particular kind of illness or disease with which the visiting man has had a great deal of experience. You can discuss your case and compare it to others he has seen. There are points where your case is different from most and others where it is the same. He's seen the course of that disease many times, and you haven't. He might be able to offer very good suggestions for therapy that you don't know about, but this is not what you really get from a visit. What he does is help you learn about the illness and disease, not about medicine in general. I think the bulk of medicine that you learn as an intern, that is, the practical information you need to take care of patients,

is drilled into you by residents and other house officers. [June 18, 1965]

The advantage of having visiting rounds with a physician specializing in a particular disease is, of course, that it affords an opportunity to learn a great deal about that one disease. Interns, then, learn by vicariously sharing a specialist's experience with his particular area of medicine. On the other hand, if a specialist dwells too much on one disease, interns can grow tired of learning what he knows.

> Freeman walked into the laboratory to find out if anyone had admitted a new patient that would be an interesting case to present to Moge, the visiting physician. No one had admitted anyone of particular interest during the night, but a student had had a patient die and thought she would make an interesting case. Freeman said, "Well, she's interesting, but I don't know." The student told him that Moge was up on her problems, and Freeman nodded and said, "Okay, why don't you present her."
>
> He turned to Rubin, the intern on his ward, and told him they would not be presenting Rubin's patient to Moge. Rubin asked, "Why not? I'm tired of hearing about cardiology. All month long I've heard about cardiology." I asked what was wrong with cardiology, and Rubin told me, "These damn visits know only their specialty. We're supposed to become rounded physicians, but these guys don't know anything beyond their specialty. How are you going to become a rounded physician? I'm not kidding. I am tired of these guys who know nothing else." He turned and walked away. Freeman told me it wasn't that bad and it might be an interesting session with Moge. [June 21, 1965]

The fact that visiting rounds are for the benefit of medical students also makes them less interesting for interns and residents.

> I don't like the philosophy of visiting rounds here. Here they are to give the students a chance to present to the visit, which is all right. But I think we frequently hear about cases that are not that interesting. I think the visiting time could be much better used by going to the problem cases on the ward and trying to get sophisticated opinions on them. On rare

occasions, if there is a really interesting case, the intern will present it. Visiting rounds are for students. In the course of time, we [interns] learn some very valuable and interesting things, but not always are they the problems on the wards. [June 22, 1965]

Students are responsible for preparing and presenting most patients for discussion during visiting rounds. Most often, however, the patients are actually picked by the interns and the resident. As one might expect, students wisely accept the patients the interns and residents select. Usually the selection of an appropriate patient is enough to make for interesting visiting rounds. Given a chance, physicians with extensive experience are able to find something interesting to say, unless the student has thoroughly covered the topic. For that reason interns assist students in preparing their presentations.

I asked Midlander [medical student] what he had learned [from interns] in the last month. "A lot of little tricks of the trade." I asked what he had learned about presenting a patient. He told me, "The first time I presented a patient, I didn't know what the visit wanted, but you learn, and you get to know what is and what isn't important. I've learned not to present everything. Always leave something for the visit to find. At first I was always pressed because the visit would ask me this and that, what he wants other people to know about the patient. Now I just present that."

"Why," I asked, "do you leave something for the visit to find?" "If you don't," he answered, "then he is pressed for something to say and gets a little touchy. Even if I have all the consults in and I know everything about the patient, I always hold back until after the visit has his say." [June 29, 1964]

Visiting rounds of the sort described below move interns, students, and residents to take steps that, hopefully, provide plenty of content for discussion.

Schooler [intern] was presenting, and Murphy (student] was holding the X-rays for the patient. Schooler described the patient as a 65-year-old male admitted for the second time and gave the results of his examination, tests, and consults [with specialists]. When he had finished, Maxwell, the visiting physician, looked at him and asked, "Well, what's the problem?" Schooler looked around, smiling at Jordan [senior resident]. Maxwell asked a couple of questions about the results of tests, and Schooler, referring to the patient's chart, gave the answers.

Murphy was looking at the X-rays, and the assistant resident, seeing him, said, "The X-rays are interesting and might be of help." He handed them to Maxwell, who turned toward the window to look at them, then said, "I agree. It's acute congestive failure." After a period of silence, he continued: "We can rule out viral infection, as well as any other possible difficulties. It should be treated as congestive failure." There was more silence. I made a note to ask Schooler why this patient had been selected for presentation.

Jordan, the senior resident, asked Maxwell what he thought of trachea punctures with a needle, to introduce a fine spray of saline. Maxwell: "I'm for it. It's fine if we had someone to do it. Hopefully, we will have someone to do it next year; I'm in favor of it, but not by everyone and everybody." In the medical history of the patient presented had been the fact that he had been asthmatic for 12 years, but that the asthma remitted and he began smoking. Schooler asked, "To get away from the subject for a while, is there any explanation for remitted asthma?" Maxwell said all he knew was that if it doesn't remit, the patient dies. The group laughed. The rounds dragged. I had the feeling that the patient wasn't exactly an exciting one and that the interns, assisted by the assistant resident and the senior resident, were trying to kill me.

It was about 11:45. Maxwell had looked at his watch a number of times before, but now he nodded and started to get up. No one said a word. He got up and started to leave. People stood, but no one said anything but the senior resident, who thanked him. Maxwell nodded and left. The assistant resident said something to the senior resident as Schooler and I started toward them. Schooler said to the senior resident, "Yes, why did you want that patient presented, Dr. Jordan?" The three of them laughed and Jordan asked, "Who did we have that was better?" [July 28, 1964]

Only four and a half hours each week are spent on visiting rounds, but interns, students and the resident must prepare carefully if those hours are to be worthwhile. The visiting physician does not prepare a lecture or other teaching materials. He simply walks onto the ward and responds to patients and their problems with opinions and examples from his own clinical experience. If he has had little experience with the patients and problems presented him, visiting rounds are merely an occasion for him to confirm what the interns and students already know. This being so, interns, students, and residents accept the responsibility for making rounds interesting. In fact, they base their actions before and during rounds on the assumption that a good visiting physician is made and not born. The way visiting physicians are handled is discussed in Chapter 8.

Interns, students, and residents need some knowledge about the visiting physician before they try to influence him. Their anticipation of his response to the presentations determine which patients are selected and how. This knowledge, then, determines the content and direction of teaching on the wards. No matter who the visiting physician may be, they want him to be interesting and their approach to him is calculated to obtain information about illness and disease in his specialty. They do not, however, want more information than they think they need. Thus, the interns and others on the wards not only partake of but attempt to control the academic activities of the internship year.

Interns spend an additional six and a half hours each week attending lectures and conferences. In addition, they spend an hour and a half every other week making chief's rounds, which do not differ in format from visiting rounds. Another four and a half hours are scheduled for consultation rounds, held by staff members of the various research divisions and affiliated clinics of the Thorndike Memorial Laboratory. Interns are expected to attend these specialty conferences, which focus on particular areas of medicine. In a month interns are scheduled to spend approximately thirty hours listening to discussions of pertinent research, diagnostic procedures, and the more recent treatments.

Interns do little more than attend this sort of activity. They do not select patients, collate laboratory results, obtain X-rays, or arrange the numerous other things they must do when presenting patients at visiting rounds. The fact that they have little to say about the content of consultation rounds, clinical pathological conferences, and such activities gives them a low opinion of their value:

> Conferences are held, I think, for the people who give conferences. It's work for them, and they feel great about it. They think they're really doing something important. They sit down the night before, get a little nervous, and write. They construct something. They build their talk. The next day, they know what they're going to say and deliver it and they think it's great. I'd love to do it. It's almost like teaching, and they probably benefit the most. But it does get repetitious. I think somebody delivering the CPC [clinical pathological conference] gets more out of delivering it than somebody in the audience listening to it. Maybe that's why we have so many conferences, because people like to give conferences. [December 23, 1964]

Although interns are not required to prepare for most academic activities, they must attend them. When attendance drops off, they are reminded that these are considered an important part of the intern year. The Schedule of Conferences and Consultation for December 1964, for example, carried the following note: "All full-time and those part-time members of the Harvard Medical Unit on duty at the hospital are expected to attend the Friday noon conferences and the Combined Services Conference." All in all, interns at Boston City Hospital are expected to participate in twenty-odd hours of visiting rounds and to attend another thirty hours of conferences, meetings, and other events each month.

SUMMARY

The work that was required of interns I observed was determined by the hospital's purpose to provide patient care, and interns spent almost all their time attending patients in emergency rooms, at clinics, and on the wards. Though the actual operation of an internship program was the responsibility of physicians and not administrators, physicians did little more than supervise the work interns had to do as employees of the hospital. This is not to say that interns do not learn, nor that physicians operating internship programs do not make an effort to provide relevant, educational experiences. Rather, it is to say that an internship is less the educational experience it is thought to be and more a job at a hospital.

When physicians admit medical school graduates for internships, they are also in fact recruiting employees for the hospital. By operating an internship program, the Harvard Medical Unit assures that the hospital's purpose to provide patient care will be accomplished, and thereby maintains itself as a part of the hospital and a segment of the medical elite. The continued operations of the hospital and the Unit depend on obtaining medical school graduates who, for whatever reason, are willing to devote that time and effort to patient care.

What I have attempted to do in this chapter is to describe the job that interns have as employees of the hospital. When interns accept the job and satisfactorily do the work of an internship, they are of course assuring their own advancement toward a medical career, including, at this hospital, the careers of the medical elite.

6. Learning the Work of an Internship

THE HARVARD Medical Unit's elite status affects the work of interns at Boston City Hospital. The primary purpose of elite segments as I have defined them is neither teaching nor patient service but medical research. The Unit can only retain its place among the elite as long as it maintains intellectual superiority, and that requires continued devotion to medical research. This is not to say that the physicians of the Harvard Medical Unit are not interested in teaching, but that they consider it less important than their other work. Though all physicians of the Harvard Medical Unit take part in the training program, they also conduct their own research and are not readily available to interns and residents. Even if they were more accessible, much of their research is not particularly helpful to the intern in his main task of working up and taking care of patients. Of course the investigations are pertinent to the problems of patients, but few research results are immediately applicable as therapy.

Since the physicians of the Harvard Medical Unit have only a limited amount of time to devote to teaching, their contact with interns is limited to conferences, lectures, and occasional consultations on the wards. In their actual work interns receive little, if any, help from Harvard physicians. They do, however, need help if they are to do the work of an internship. Interns must learn how to do the work that is assigned them or they will fail to be valuable employees and, by failing, impede the delivery of patient care, subvert the Unit's place in the hospital, and make it impossible to accomplish whatever purposes they themselves may have in serving internships. The purpose of this chapter is to describe how interns learn to do their work as employees and how they learn to maximize the return on their investment of time and effort in this work.

Interns arrive at the hospital with some knowledge of what their work will be. They have learned a great deal from books, lectures, conferences, and clinical work at medical school. How to do the work of an internship, however, is something they must learn from others, not from the physicians who are responsible for their training but busy with other work. They are faced with the initial problem of learning the ropes. But there are no teachers of the ropes, only busy medical scientists. Who, if not Harvard physicians, are their teachers?

LEARNING THE ROPES [1]

Newcomers in any social situation go through an initial process of learning the ropes: finding out who the other people in that situation are, where they are located, what they do, what they expect the newcomer to do, and how they want him to do it. We seldom dignify this process by calling it learning. Educators may attempt to cover the kinds of things a newcomer must learn in brief orientations, but they expect everyone to make an

1. The following section first appeared, in most part, as "Learning the Ropes: Situational Learning in Four Occupational Training Programs" by Blanche Geer, Jack Haas, Charles V. Vona, Stephen J. Miller, Clyde Woods, and Howard S. Becker in *Among the People*, I. Deutscher and E. J. Thompson (eds.), (New York, Basic Books, 1968), pp. 223–228.

adjustment to the school, the hospital, or any other organization. When newcomers adjust successfully, no one thinks anything more about this part of their learning experience. But newcomers who do not learn the ropes are likely to get the attention of those people in charge of their education.

Sociologists, however, have long been interested in successful situational learning.[2] Let us examine the process of initial learning on the Harvard Medical Services at Boston City Hospital.

After a short meeting at which the physicians, nurses, and other hospital personnel are introduced, the intern goes to the wards or clinics to which he is assigned. He supposedly is ready to do his work. Actually, however, he must successfully negotiate the process of initial learning in order to do what is expected of him and before he can initiate any other kind of learning.

The intern begins his training in a familiar environment. He has been in hospitals before and has some idea of what interns do. He comes to his new duties with the confidence of a good medical school record, without which he would not be in the Harvard program, and the newly acquired authority of a medical degree.

He enters a highly differentiated hierarchy of medical and hospital personnel, each group a potential source of situational learning. He does not begin at the bottom of the total hospital structure, but immediately fills the central position accorded a physician. Students, nurses, and other hospital personnel are his subordinates; patients, in his immediate care. In the hierarchy of physicians, he ranks beneath the assistant resident, who supervises his work and was himself an intern only the year before. Above the assistant residents are senior residents, a chief resident, the program director, and research and consulting physicians.

The intern has a clearly identifiable peer group. The sixteen admitted to the program each year, though a small number, have the advantage of being a cohort who pass the year together.

2. For example, Donald Roy, "Quota Restriction and Goldbricking in the Machine Shop," *American Journal of Sociology,* 57 (March, 1952), pp. 427–442; Donald R. Cressey, ed., *The Prison* (New York, Holt, Rinehart and Winston, 1961); and Erving Goffman, *Asylums: Essays on the Social Situation of Mental Patients and Other Inmates* (Garden City, Doubleday, 1961).

Furthermore, they see one another frequently during rounds, in the laboratory, and at conferences and meals.[3]

From the outset, superiors encourage the intern to define his chief responsibility as getting his work done. His work is caring for patients. Getting it done, however, is not just a matter of performing a series of tasks. He must base his diagnoses on information provided by other hospital personnel, as well as on what he himself discovers. The treatment he prescribes may be carried out by still others. He must have the cooperation of others in running tests, taking X-rays, and getting medical consultation. Since in many respects his job is administrative, he must learn to manage people so that events proceed rapidly and in proper sequence.

At the beginning of his internship the new man faces a number of problems, some of which result from the ambiguity of being both the physician in charge and a neophyte with much to learn. He carries out his duties under the eyes of the assistant resident and other physicians—men whose good opinion he needs. At the same time he is in the somewhat uncomfortable position of having to learn from students, nurses, and other staff who lack the authority of a degree in medicine but who know the ropes at BCH.

> Field said, "On my ward, I'd be lost without my student. He just took over. There I was. I didn't even know what forms to fill out, but he did. He didn't have to, but he filled the forms out and really helped me out. I wouldn't know what the hell to do if it wasn't for the students on the floor." [June 27, 1964]

Where forms are kept, which ones to use, and the niceties of filling them out are administrative details the intern must learn if his work is to go smoothly. Nevertheless, they are details—not the kind of information a man wants to bother his superiors

3. For discussion of the consequences of admission in cohorts, see Howard S. Becker, "Personal Change in Adult Life," *Sociometry*, 27 (March, 1964), pp. 40–53; on irregular admission see Stanton Wheeler, "The Structure of Formally Organized Socialization Settings," in *Socialization After Childhood*, S. Wheeler and O. G. Brim (New York, John Wiley, 1966), pp. 53–113.

for—and students are a convenient source of such information.[4]
Nurses teach other ropes, often crucial for the care of patients.

> [The patient's] feet were uncovered; they were horribly scaled
> and dirty; the nails had been allowed to grow and become
> twisted and gnarled. Andrew turned to me and said, "That's
> the way witches must look. I think it's just dirt and failure to
> cut those nails. We'll have to have someone look at it. It's
> interesting, though." We returned to the ward kitchen. Andrew
> mentioned the woman's feet to the nurse. In response to his
> question about scissors with which to cut the toenails, the
> nurse said, "Oh no! Don't do that. Put in for a consult with
> Dr. B. in the diabetic clinic. He's the foot man. The only one
> around. He'll come and use a saw." [July 7, 1964]

Thus the nurse saved the intern from possible error, and gave
him two pieces of situational data. First, he learned something
of the limits of his responsibility: In this hospital interns need
not perform a procedure that entails risk of infection for the
diabetic patient. Second, to his growing fund of administrative
facts he added a name (Dr. B.), a place (the diabetic clinic),
and a procedural arrangement (consultation).

The intern does not always find nurses so helpful. He soon
begins to recognize how much he depends on them to carry out
the treatment he orders.

> I heard Andrew say to Holt, "I'll tell you, the nurses can
> make your internship hell." "How?" I asked. Andrew replied,
> "Well, they just won't do things for you if you don't handle
> them right. You have to flirt a little, never appear heavy-
> handed, and just jolly them along." I asked, "Do you mean
> that if you don't do this, they won't do the things they have
> to for you?" Heath [medical student] said, "I think they just
> won't do anything for you." Holt nodded and Andrew said,
> "That's right. If you want to make things easy on yourself, you
> have to get the nurse on your side." [July 27, 1964]

4. This information is not needed, of course, by those who were at
BCH as students. For full discussion of the overlapping student-intern
rotation, see Stephen J. Miller, "Training of a Physician," a paper read
at the annual meeting of the Midwest Sociological Society, 1965.

For these interns at least, learning to manage nurses is part of learning the ropes.

The intern also learns the ropes from the assistant resident, who makes himself almost continuously available. During rounds, when they are together at the bedside, he tells interns about important hospital policies on the treatment of various diseases, explaining them and outlining the steps to follow in carrying them out. It is the assistant resident who tells the intern how to integrate sequences of medical treatment with administrative rules in order to avoid delays.

> The first patient had been admitted in coma, Andrew had stayed up with her most of the night. Wilson [assistant resident] said, "I think she's coming around. When she does come around all the way, I see no need for the IV. You can start her eating. When she is eating, just call the executive office and take her off the danger list. You can't discharge them right from the danger list. If it's at night, call the main desk and let them know." [July 27, 1964]

Thinking ahead so that medical contingencies and hospital regulations do not conflict is one of the important things an intern must master.

He makes more progress toward control of his work by the process interns call "running around."

> Rodney said, "Let's go over to X-ray and see if we can't squeeze these pictures in." We walked across the roofs and entered the basement of the building. Rodney had two, a gall bladder and a GI [gastrointestinal] series. Joe, a fellow in a lab coat, asked, "Is it an emergency? Do you want the pictures right away?" Rodney said, "I'd like to get them as soon as possible, but it's not an emergency." Joe said, "Well, follow me; you have to put it in the book then. If it's something you want done right away, or it's an emergency, then either see the nurse or myself."
> He then led us around the corner, where two officious-looking young men in white shirts with ties and dark trousers were seated with a pile of ledgers between them. The fellow behind the desk asked, "Is that right? Is that the way you want it done? The GI first, then the gall bladder?" Rodney said, "That's

not my preference. I just want to get the pictures taken as soon as possible." The fellow behind the desk said, "Well, that's the way it's usually done. We do the GI first, then the gall bladder." He began thumbing through his ledgers. He assigned the GI for the next day. Joe said, "Well, maybe you'll be able to get the bladder done the day after. Good luck." He left.

The fellow behind the desk said, "I don't know about the gall bladder." Rodney asked, "What about the next day, isn't it free?" The fellow thumbed through the ledger again, never letting us see the date and said, "No, there's no way of getting her in. We're just booked solid. There is no other time before next week. The barium doesn't clear out that quickly anyway." Rodney shrugged his shoulders and agreed to the dates. We left and he said, "There's a hell of a lot of running around you have to do here." [July 7, 1964]

Thus, by encouraging him to follow certain schedules and routines, hospital employees train the intern in what, in their view, is the proper performance of his duties.[5]

In the beginning you think you really have to do things that way, and you do everything hospital employees tell you to. How the hell do you know what's what? But now, I think I know how to get what I want.

In time, the intern learns to handle these situations. By understanding work that lies outside his area of responsibility but is directly related to his own efforts, he increases the possibility of controlling the sequences of his work.

In a relatively short time the intern grows familiar with his new situation. His central position gives him access to a variety of sources of information. The prestige of his medical degree may well ease his dealing with some groups, but it sometimes fosters ambiguity by suggesting that he already knows the ropes he is trying to learn. His previous education may have fitted him to manage his patients medically, but he still has to demonstrate that he can handle his administrative responsibilities.

The intern could turn to the assistant resident for all the infor-

5. For relevant analysis, see David Mechanic, "Sources of Power of Lower Participants," *Administrative Science Quarterly,* 7 (December, 1962), pp. 349–364.

mation he needs, but he does not. Instead, he accepts teaching from each group whose work intersects his. Learning about their work at first hand, he builds personal relationships that facilitate his own. As interaction continues, he learns how to joke with nurses and negotiate with technicians to secure their cooperation. So much of his work is managerial that he must understand other groups in order to achieve a measure of control over them and over events.

Learning the ropes is not simply a matter of acquiring facts about people, places, and things. It is also a matter of learning how to deal with them successfully. All interns must take the same first steps. Success entails the mastery of skills apparently unrelated to graduate training in medicine.

The intern, like all newcomers to any situation, must make a social map of his surroundings and relate the actions of others to his own. Although he is unlikely to formulate his ideas clearly unless action presents problems, he nevertheless defines his situation and acts on the definition. He seeks out those groups whose work affects his own in order to learn their habits and circumvent delays.

Peers, subordinates, auxiliary personnel—in fact, any frequent contact—may become sources of situational learning. Moreover, interns are capable of considerable ingenuity in finding teachers. If those who should teach them are not available, they turn to peers; if peers are unavailable, they use subordinates. Supplied with both superiors and subordinates, they tactfully exploit them all. Evidently they know that failure to learn the ropes may preclude learning anything else. If the intern does not learn whom to consult and how to secure his help, he will not learn what the consulting physician can teach him about medicine. If he does not learn to get on with his fellows, they will not teach him what they may have learned, and he may not discover important things about how to do his work.

If the capacity for situational learning is distinct from that for ordinary learning, as it may be, interns and others who fail in training may do so because they have not learned the ropes, which involves techniques seldom included in the program of training.

SUCCESSION AND TEACHING THE ROPES [6]

A fact of the teaching hospital's organization is that people periodically vacate the positions they have had, and other people come in to fill the vacancies. Interns arrive at the hospital about the same time each year and leave, or at least vacate their positions as interns, at the end of the year. Almost simultaneously, new interns arrive, supposedly ready to do their jobs.

At the time of succession there is little time for orientation or indoctrination. The work on the wards and clinics goes on. There is no way to halt the hospital's operations until the newcomers have learned the ropes. The intern, much like any new worker, is introduced to the techniques of getting things done as he comes face-to-face with the problems and duties of his job.[7] How, then, do interns learn what problems face them and what their duties are? Since no one is designated to teach them these things, are they allowed simply to go their own way? This is, in fact, how they do learn a great deal. But interns left entirely on their own would disrupt hospital routine. Therefore, the training program must be set up so that succession can take place with a minimum of difficulty. Though all interns must take the same beginning steps, training programs may make those steps easy or difficult.

A member of studies show how occupational groups with permanent positions in organizations prepare people who are entering to stay for a short time.[8] But university or university-affiliated hospitals are somewhat unusual organizations, in that many people hold only temporary positions. Students, interns, and residents, whose work is similar, come and go regularly. They are not making careers at the hospital, but are spending

6. The following section first appeared as part of "Exchange and Negotiated Learning in Graduate Medical Education," by Stephen J. Miller in the *Sociological Quarterly* (Fall, 1966).

7. Joseph Bensman and Israel Gerver, "Crime and Punishment in the Modern Factor," in Alvin W. Gouldner and others, eds., *Modern Sociology* (New York, Harcourt, Brace and World, 1963).

8. I am indebted to Robert S. Weiss for much information on this matter. Cf. his *Processes of Organization* (Ann Arbor, University of Michigan, 1956).

time there as a contingency of future careers. An orderly succession of people in temporary positions would be further facilitated by arrangements that would permit them to orient one another.

Most assistant residents at the Harvard Medical Services were interns the previous year. When they move up, they become responsible for the administration of a ward, which includes responsibility for the adjustment of interns. The assistant resident, having only yesterday been an intern himself, knows the ropes and what it is to learn them. Assistant residents teach new interns a great deal about the traditions of the medical services and the hospital's ways of doing things. They are valuable sources of information because they have successfully passed through situations the beginners have yet to meet and manage.

Students from the Harvard Medical School come to BCH to obtain experience with patients. They come every few months and a cohort of students arrive a month before new interns arrive, at a time when departing interns are looking forward to residencies, either here or somewhere else. By now these interns look upon most of their work as routine, not as the challenge they first found it to be. They are, in other words, ready to delegate much of their work to other willing hands. Medical students, eager for experience and a chance to exercise responsibility, accept all the work the interns give them.

Although a great deal of work is delegated to students at this time, they are not empowered to exercise much discretion. They are supervised by and must defer to interns. Thus students learn acceptable performance. They do, in fact, adopt many of the interns' maneuvers and procedures. Shortly before new interns arrive, as a consequence of the time of the year, medical students are allowed, to some extent, to take the role of the interns. They thus gain valuable information about the way things work at the hospital, information that new interns also need.

The ones in the best position to teach newcomers the ropes are not, as we might assume, those who have been at the hospital for a long time, but students who have been there only a month and assistant residents, who have been there a year. The students stay for a few months; they arrive a month before succession takes place and leave a month after new interns come to the hospital. Their work is similar to that of interns. Through their ward and clinic assignments they will come in contact with interns every day, and they can help interns without disrupting the routine of the hospital, because they need not stop what they are doing.

THE PROCESS OF SUCCESSION

Not every intern is a newcomer to Boston City Hospital. A few have been there as students. At the time of succession, interns who were students last year are assigned the duties of night float or are placed on call on the wards. At least a few of the incoming interns, then, may be used to assure that work continues without interruption. Interns who were students at the hospital have an advantage that some of them use to facilitate succession.

> In the lab there were three wire baskets on a desk, each containing patient charts and labeled with the name of an intern. There were only a few charts in Cooper's basket. Wallace [assistant resident] was standing next to me. I pointed to the basket and said, "Cooper must be a lucky boy not to have too much to do today." Wallace replied, "Cooper has an advantage because he knows how to get his work done quickly. He has nodded and replied, "Yes, he was a medical student here." managed to keep ahead of things and not get behind." I asked if he had this advantage because he knew the ropes. Wallace [August 24, 1964]

Late the same day I asked Cooper about his work:

> "Do you like working on the wards?" Cooper replied, "Well, it's not new. I was here as a medical student not too long ago, so I've been on the wards before." I asked him if having been a medical student at the hospital helped when he first came as an intern. Cooper: "And how! The tradition here is to have the interns who were last on as students be night float. The night float is on his own, a step up from being a medical

student. There's no one to watch over your shoulder, and you take care of everything. I'm sure that's why they pick us to be night float first, because we know what's what."

Apparently those in authority do recognize that new interns must make some adjustments before their work can progress smoothly. At the beginning of the year, they make succession somewhat less difficult. Even so, all the problems are not resolved. Other interns must still learn the ropes before they can also do their work quickly and properly.

Interns entirely new to the situation depend on those who have information. They depend on the medical students and the assistant residents. Students have already completed half their two-month assignment and are now available to teach those who are usually thought of as teaching them. ·

> When I entered the laboratory, Barrow [intern] had a bottle of urine in his hand. Daily [student] was at a microscope. Barrow in a loud voice asked: "What do I do now? Oh, I wish I had someone to help me with this." He then poured the urine into test tubes. Daily walked over to Barrow, who asked, "And what do we use for testing pH?" Daily handed him a bottle of litmus paper. Barrow said, "Oh, you use this here. We didn't use these at _____. As a matter of fact, I prefer these [reaching up to a shelf for a bottle of pills]. These are much better." Barrow then put mixed urine and water in a test tube and dropped in a pill, with Daily watching him all the time.
>
> Barrow shook the test tube and, holding it up to the light, said: "There, that's a good color and tells you everything you need to know." He then repeated the urine test, using the paper strips Daily had handed him. He said to Daily: "You see, now look. What can you tell from that?" Daily shook his head and said, "But you are supposed to read the sugar first. The rest you can read any time." Barrow then measured the urine and used the paper to do his tests, then turned to Daily and asked, "It is 64, isn't it?" Daily said it was, and Barrow left the laboratory. [June 29, 1964]

Thus the intern learned from the student the hospital's way

to do a urinalysis. The student, because of his experience, had the advantage over the new intern.

Since the student has this advantage, he can continue taking the role of 'an intern. A relationship of this sort between the student and new interns continues for almost, but not quite, all the rest of the student's stay at the hospital. There comes a time when the new intern has learned his way around and no longer needs to incur the indignity of student infringement on his work. The exchange of information has reduced the student's advantage and interns have less to gain by permitting them to intrude.

Students, having been given a good deal of autonomy, resent and resist the intern's attempts to regain control of their relationship. What is apparently a cooperative relationship can become antagonistic.

> Kennedy [student] and I walked to my car. I said, "You can never win with Harry [intern]." Kennedy said, "Yes, but he's going to be told off in a couple of days. The other students will tell him off too." When I asked him what he meant, he replied, "Well, we're a spoiled bunch of medical students. The other interns allowed us to take a lot of the responsibility for patients. We didn't have to do much scut work. Now these guys have been a lot rougher and ask us to do a lot more of it."
>
> I told him that I had spent the last two days with the interns he was talking about, and that Harry had told MacDonald [another student] to take his day off, that he would do MacDonald's work. Kennedy said, "Oh, well Harry shouldn't have done that. MacDonald should do his own work, and Harry should do his." I said that I didn't actually know it was MacDonald's work. I told Kennedy I thought Harry forgot it was MacDonald's day off, and when he remembered, told MacDonald to forget the work because Harry would do it. Kennedy said, "Well, we have been doing a lot of their scut work." [June 29, 1964]

This student did not resent having to do scut work so much as he minded having less responsibility for patients. Students expect to do scut; that is, menial and routine chores. The question of responsibility, however, is a potential ground for conflict when the interns first arrive. The assistant resident will, of course, resolve any disputes in favor of the intern. The possibility of conflict, however, exists until the student leaves the hospital at the end of his tour at the hospital. Students who come after them will from the start be subordinate to interns and depend on them, as interns had previously depended on students, to teach them the ropes.

The initial problem of situational learning requires an intern to determine his course of action on the spot, as problems arise and his duties are made clear to him. For the same reason that he at first accepts medical students as peers, he accepts the assistant resident as his superior. It is the intern's dependence on the assistant resident as a source of information, rather than the authority vested in him, that determines their relationship.

The assistant resident, however, is also facing new problems and attempting to meet the demands of a new job. Why should he take the time and trouble to teach the ropes to interns? What does he have to gain? For one thing, his work is facilitated by his having influence as well as authority over interns. Since interns depend on him, he can define an acceptable level and direction of effort without resorting to authority. By tactfully exploiting their dependence, he can control the way interns discharge their duties without raising questions about their supposed autonomy.

> I told Greenberg, an assistant resident, that I had read that at one university hospital interns do not immediately get put in charge of patients. The article said that's something you have to earn by demonstrating your competence; and even then, a lot depends on the resident. Greenberg said, "Well, the philosophy here is different from that. The interns are the patients' doctors from the very beginning, and from the first day that they arrive, they are the doctors. The assistant resident sits back. He doesn't abdicate responsibility, but at the same time, he doesn't do the work. This is probably the best way because in a very short time interns become confident, more confident than if they had people making their decisions for them. This doesn't mean that people aren't around all the time

to help make the decisions. I think that this place is as good as it is because there are always assistant residents around who have been through it all and can give you the right kind of guidance and leadership if you have problems you can't handle." [December 15, 1964]

The same conversation illustrates the part that assistant residents, exercising their influence over interns, play in the process of succession.

I asked Greenberg what he thought was a good intern. He replied, "You know that the guys who come here are intelligent, and you assume that all of them are good from the start. The really good interns are those who have the right attitude and the willingness to work, and to me, it's as simple as that." Miller: "What do you mean by the right attitude?" Greenberg explained: "The interns who are really good are those who go and get the work done. If an intern starts by going home and reading the journals the night before so he can come back and look smart all around, people sort of, you know, let him know immediately that this is just not the way things are done." I asked him why it wasn't that way, and he replied:

"Well, I don't know. I never have been able to figure it out, but it is the spirit that is sort of passed down from generation to generation. People exchange information, but not to impress each other. Nobody jumps on you because you don't know exactly how to treat asthma or you don't know how to treat cirrhosis. They just tell you how in a nice way. When I was on the male ward [during the first month of internship] the boys really just didn't know how to approach a patient. You had to sort of be right on top of things and say to them, Now, let's get two blood cultures, or the patient may need this or that. Then you tell them how it's done. You have to say to them, 'Well, I really think we ought to do this on the guy.' They get the point and they listen. You don't have to say, 'Do two blood cultures.' Now [later in the year] they're asking why it should be done. At the beginning so much of what they learn is information passed on from year to year. Interns assume it's good information because good people tell them to do it that way. For example, if [a Harvard professor] tells us that X is much better than Y, then we figure it is. If we hear that when we're interns, when we become assistant residents, we pass it down to the new interns. So much of the internship here is learning what has been done before and what is considered good practice by the group ahead of you."

Besides increasing his influence, helping to break in new interns gives the assistant resident the satisfaction of training successors. His efforts also earn him the regard of interns, which supports his claim to authority.

The particular conditions of the initial relationship between intern and assistant residents, like those between interns and students, do not persist through the year. The intern gains experience, the same kinds of experience for which he values the assistant resident, and this in turn makes him less amenable to control. There comes a time when interns consider themselves competent to make decisions on their own. By then they have their own standards and a plan of action for making sure their patients receive proper medical attention.

Despite this new independence, interns are still influenced by assistant residents. The latter part of the year finds them looking forward to their own residencies. Needless to say, it would not be politic for them to deny the authority of positions they themselves will soon occupy.

The end of the year is also the time when interns will again tolerate student infringement on their work. By this time they feel they have gained as much experience as they can on this job, so they have nothing to lose by delegating some of their responsibility. Thus another group of students is prepared to teach another group of new interns the ropes. The process of succession will begin again.

The process of succession is not so much a critical aspect of training as it is the means by which physicians free themselves of the tasks of orienting interns and supervising their work at the hospital. If the Unit's purpose was first and foremost training, it could be assumed that Harvard physicians would be teachers of the ropes and, further, responsible for overseeing the work of interns. The internship is, of course, a period of training, but to assume it is nothing more would overlook the character of the medical elite.

The Unit must provide patient care without obligating the time of its physicians who have other and, if the Unit is to regain its place among the elite, more important things to do. Physicians who are busy conducting research have little time to devote to routine patient care. They also have little time to devote to teaching interns the ropes of patient care. The processes of succession and situational learning allow the Unit to prepare and use interns to provide patient care without unnecessarily interrupting the research and other activities of Harvard physicians.

7. Social Exchange and Dynamics of Work

THE HARVARD Medical Unit exists at the hospital because its interns do the work that must be done to provide patient care. I have described the work and how interns learn to do it in preceding chapters. My purpose in this chapter is to describe what they learn to do to be successful interns.

Interns learn that to provide patient care and accomplish some of their own purposes as well, they must make deals to obtain the cooperation of the people with whom they must work. Making deals facilitates the doing of the work and assures satisfactory performance as an intern. A satisfactory performance obtains the good will of Harvard physicians, which is necessary to assure future opportunities for attractive medical careers.

The deals that interns must make are actually social exchanges. Social exchange may be briefly defined as the obligation incurred by a recipient of something valuable to reciprocate, when the occasion arises, by furnishing his benefactor with something of equal value. The relationship between interns and medical students during succession is one of social exchange. Students anxious for experience and responsibility were permitted to take the role of intern in exchange for information interns had to have if they were to do their work. Other relationships may also be analyzed as processes by which hospital personnel negotiate the exchange of information, goods, or services.

A relationship of this sort begins when one person benefits by the acts of another and reciprocates adequately, thus inducing the other person to continue the relationship under conditions that are mutually satisfactory. The relationship is a product of the beneficial and reciprocal actions of two or more people, and will persist as long as the people involved are more or less equally rewarded. The internship consists of numerous sets of such exchange relationships.

When interns begin their year at the hospital, they have little idea of what is actually expected of them. No one tells them the rules, nor how they are to work with other people. Since they must work together with people, they evolve, through social exchange, a network of relationships that serves as a rudimentary social structure.[1] Social structure, in these terms, is a network of relationships made up of social exchanges.[2] The social structure of the services of the Harvard Medical Unit grows out of exchanges between interns and the people with whom they have to work: other interns and residents, physicians, nurses, and ancillary hospital personnel. These people who come together negotiate relationships that facilitate their work. The relationship between interns and students, for example, is not so much prescribed by the hospital's normative patterns as it is negotiated by the participants. Each year interns must negotiate mutually satisfactory relationships, not only with students but also with a

1. The "rudimentary structure" consists of informal relationships and unofficial norms, which are evolved within the formal organization of the medical setting. For a further discussion of "rudimentary structure" see Peter M. Blau, *Exchange and Power* (New York, John Wiley, 1964), pp. 92–93.
2. Social structure in these terms is also discussed by William J. Goode, "A Theory of Role Strain," *American Sociological Review*, 25, 4 (August, 1960) particularly pp. 494–495.

variety of other people. These relationships, far from being idiosyncratic, are consistent patterns characteristic of the organization of the Unit at Boston City Hospital.[3]

SOCIAL EXCHANGE AND NEGOTIATED LEARNING

Interns on the Harvard Medical Services work in the shadow of the Thorndike Medical Laboratory, whose staff includes many distinguished medical scientists. Many other physicians are studying specialties or working on research projects at BCH. These physicians constitute an enviable pool of expert opinion in almost every field of medicine. Working with men of such caliber is considered one of the benefits of a university internship. It is essential to realize, however, that the work of interns and the interests of medical scientists and specialists sometimes conflict. The patients whom interns care for are not always interesting to other physicians. Interns have much to gain by drawing on the knowledge of these physicians, but teaching and consulting offer few rewards to scientists and specialists. They have their own work to do, and tend to resist other demands on their time. This is not to say that the Harvard physicians do not do any teaching or consulting; but they do control their investment of time in these activities and try to make the consultation and teaching more satisfying to themselves.

The Harvard physicians teach because they take pride in training the young men who will become their colleagues and eventually their successors. "Not everyone," one of them remarked, "has the chance to shape the men who will be practicing medicine." Those who provide information when it is needed also earn the regard of interns. "It's a good feeling to have [interns] look up to you for advice," another physician said. But these rewards are not always payment enough for the time and effort that teaching and consulting require. "Sure you have an impact as a teacher, and you want to help as much as you can, but you can't get your work done that way." Most physicians

3. The government agencies observed by Peter M. Blau are other examples of structure consisting of negotiated social relationships. See *The Dynamics of Bureaucracy* (Chicago, University of Chicago Press, 1955).

try to increase their compensation by making additional demands. Most obviously, they insist on dealing with problems of some interest to them as well as of benefit to interns.

In these circumstances interns can expect Harvard physicians to teach and may further claim their assistance, but they must respond to the demands established as payment for the time and effort expended in their behalf. This means that they must negotiate their relationships with teachers and consultants. Thus they have to determine what they have to exchange in return for the information and assistance they want. Interns distinguish among the kinds of Harvard physicians they encounter. They consider visiting physicians different from consulting physicians. As one explained:

> The visiting physician should be a man with a lot of practical experience who can help you in a very real way. He should say things with the kind of confidence that can come from practicing on your own for a long time. I want the benefit of that kind of experience. He doesn't have to be a super-specialist with all the answers. The consulting physicians have all the answers because they're the smart young men of medicine. They want to do this test or they want to do that test, but the visit should say, "The patient is 92 years old; send him to a nursing home."

I asked, "Would it be fair to say that you are looking for information from both the visit and the consult, but different kinds of information?"

> Yes. Here's a good example: We've had a lot of lung disease. We have Dr. Cohn, who is an internist; his specialty is pulmonary disease. We also have an infectious disease consult, Dr. Goode. Together, they have what I want. Cohn is smart, but his attitude is one of the New England doctor, sitting back and looking over the patient. Goode, on the other hand, is a good consult, because he is interested in finding the organism responsible and treating it with the right sort of antibiotics. Cohn is the sort of man who can go up to the bedside and examine the patient, making a diagnosis in a homely sort of way. He doesn't know that much about the various organisms but he can tell you a lot about how people get lung abscesses,

what kind of abscesses he has seen, how he has treated lung abscesses, and so on. He can also tell you what you can expect to see in a day or a week with a patient like that because he has seen what has happened to other patients. The infectious disease man doesn't tell you those things. He tells you to treat it with acromycin, and it does work, but you want to know more than that. If you put a visit and a consult together, they both can teach you something about managing a patient. What you have to do is to take the visit and make him into what you want him to be. The consult is pretty much what he is, and you have to take him as he is. [February 9, 1965]

THE VISITING PHYSICIANS

Interns agree that they do not get much assistance from visiting physicians. The latter have little to say about patient care, though they are interesting for other reasons.

Let's face it, they have little to do with what goes on. They don't help us with the practical management, or with immediate problems. What they have to say is rarely pertinent to what you are doing, though they are interesting. They are most interesting when they reminisce about the cases they've had, or when they discuss the literature. They have been good for me, but not because of their help with patients. I think they're good because it has been interesting to hear about the patients they've had, or to learn about the various approaches to patients, medicine, medical education, and so forth. They are like nice, current history books.[4] [June 11, 1965]

All visiting physicians, however, are not so helpful. Interns must be careful how they manage them if their visits are to be useful. (I have described an attempt to manage the visiting physician in Chapter 5.) When presented with a patient whose problems are obvious, the visiting physician can add little to what the interns already know. He cannot reminisce nor discuss the medical literature because the patient has no problems rel-

4. Blau, *Exchange and Power*, p. 132.

evant to the visit's specialty. Since there is nothing he can say, he will bring his teaching to an end as soon as possible. Visiting rounds of this sort happen most often during the first month or so, before the interns learn how to manage a visit, before they know the conditions of their relationships with visits and how they must handle them to create a teaching situation.

All visiting physicians are, of course, willing to teach. But most do not know what they will teach until they are actually presented with patients. When a visiting physician sees a patient with problems relevant to his particular experience, he can help make the diagnosis, or he can add to what interns know by drawing on his own special knowledge. Patients with obvious problems or problems not related to his specialty do not lend themselves to teaching. Sometimes, in order to find an interesting case, a visiting physician may make a round of the ward to see for himself what patients are available.

> I arrived on the ward a few minutes after visiting rounds began and found the group making walking rounds of the patients. I asked Hertman, an intern, who decided to do this. He said, "Rand [visit] hasn't seen all the patients for a while, so he wanted to make rounds." The interns looked anything but interested in what was going on. Landfeld [intern] would, for example, look at me and hold his arms straight out with palms up, rolling his eyes up into his head and shrugging his shoulders. Hertman was carrying patient charts with him and reading them as the visit examined patients. The students and the assistant resident were discussing the patients with the visiting physician. The interns, standing off to the back of the group, had nothing to say. I asked Landfeld, "Why see the patients?" He replied, "We didn't have anyone to present, so Rand wants to know exactly what kind of patients are on the ward. He's using walking rounds as a chance to find some problems he can talk about." [May 24, 1965]

Many visiting physicians will not make the effort to find patients for themselves. On the wards for only a few hours each week to teach, visits cannot know all the patients and cannot always choose the ones with problems that lend themselves to teaching. Even those who do look for patients can do so only occasionally. But the visit must always have patients with problems related to his specialty, or his position as a teacher will be untenable. The assistant resident and the interns have the continuing responsibility to find and present suitable patients to him.

> The assistant resident, Goldson, walked into the laboratory and asked Williams, a student, if he had admitted any new patients. Williams said, "No, not today, but I had two that died yesterday." Goldson nodded and said, "That'll have to do." Williams asked, "How about that woman that died? Couldn't we do something with her?" "Well," said Goldson, "she's interesting but I don't know if Kenner, a visiting physician, is up on her problems. But why don't you present her first?" Williams said, "I don't know. I think that Benson should present her first because mine is really only a comment and won't give him much to talk about." Goldson said, "That's OK, because after you present, we will have to go down to the ward and see Benson's patient. So why don't you present first and we won't have to come back up?" Williams agreed. When Warren, an intern, came in, Goldson told him that they would present the woman who died. "Why?" asked Warren. "She died. I am tired of hearing about cardiology. All month long I've heard about cardiology."
>
> Goldson shrugged. I asked what was wrong with cardiology. Warren said, "These damn visits know only their specialty. We're supposed to become rounded physicians, but these guys don't know anything beyond their specialty. How are you going to become a rounded physician? I'm not kidding. I'm tired of these guys and how we have to handle them." Goldson shrugged again and said, "Kenner isn't that bad. He's really pretty good, and I think this patient might make for an interesting session." [June 21, 1965]

The patients selected were both suitable for teaching. The dead woman presented problems relevant to the visit's specialty, and the new admission would require a complete presentation of the history, physical examination, and laboratory results.

Since students usually present patients, arranging a successful presentation of a suitable patient requires their collaboration.

Interns teach students how to present patients so as to set the stage for teaching.

The visiting physicians know all about this process. They often make some reference to reveal that they are aware of how patients are selected and presented for their benefit.

> A male admitted with a suspected myiocardial infarct was presented by Burke, an intern, to Tower, a visiting physician. When Burke finished, Tower asked for a diagnosis. Burke said, "Infarct." The assistant resident then explained, "We frequently get cases with chest pains, negative lab results, and spurious symptoms. Are there any particular clues to watch for?" Tower smilingly replied, "You're not asking a very well-informed source." No one asked another question about diagnosis. Lynd, an intern, asked, "Do you have any strong opinions on the treatment of infarcts?" "I have no strong opinions," Tower answered, "I always listen to the house staff." Smilingly he added, "Why don't we just go on to what we can talk about?" [July 27, 1964]

The rules of this game are simple. First, residents, interns, and students must agree to accept what the visit defines as the content of his teaching. That is, they must talk about something he knows about. Second, questions must be relevant to the visit's interests, experience, or knowledge. Finally, the visit must be left with something to say. Interns, therefore, do not always make known their diagnosis or tell a visit the results of consultations. If they do, the visit has nothing much to say.

If they play the game properly, interns are rewarded with instruction. If they don't, they get little or none. When all concerned abide by the rules, the relationship is satisfactory to all.

The conditions of the exchange between interns and visiting physicians appear to cost the interns very little. In exchange for selecting and presenting suitable patients, they gain teaching performances by distinguished scientists and knowledgeable physicians. They don't, however, get off absolutely free. The most obvious additional cost is that they must make an hour and a half in a busy schedule for visiting rounds. This often takes them away from their patients and leaves them with less time to do their work, but the problem is not insoluble.

> A medical student was presenting a 65-year-old male with rheumatoid arthritis and a fever of unknown origin. I did not see either Lynd [intern] or Dickson (student) at rounds, so I went looking for them. They were working on a patient. Lynd was saying as I entered the patient's cubicle, "Your job is to take care of the patient first. There's no reason why, when you have a patient this sick, you should make visiting rounds. Your responsibility is to the patients." I would have thought that this was said for my benefit, but he had said the same thing earlier in the presence of the assistant resident, other interns, and students. When the assistant resident told them that rounds would start promptly at 10:30, Dickson had said "I'm not quite finished with my new admission." Lynd had said, "Well, if you can't finish in time, you'll just have to miss the visit. Patients come first, and you have a couple of acute problems on the ward. It's more important to [attend] them than to make visiting rounds." [July 8, 1965]

Interns expect visiting physicians to understand that they have a great deal of work to do. Obviously they are not required to attend visiting rounds when they have critical patients to care for or when there is a medical emergency. More than that, however, they expect the visit to tolerate their being late or leaving early.

> The visit [Tower] was waiting for the house staff to begin rounds. Rosenberg [intern] said to me, "In case you're wondering why I'm always late for visiting rounds, it's because I'm getting my work done." I knew he had been introducing sodium chloride into an intravenous set-up. "I'm late," he said, "and I'm sure the visit thinks I'm terrible, but he knows I have to do my work. These guys know it's not easy to get there on time. When you have so much to do, you can't sit here and listen to everything he has to say. An hour and a half is enough. That's all the time they are supposed to get and they can't ask for more. The visits have to be flexible or I won't come at all." [July 17, 1964]

Loss of time is not so annoying to interns as another price they must pay for the teaching they receive on visiting rounds. Since each particular specialist makes visiting rounds for a month, this means that all month they discuss the same or similar medical problems. Thus rounds with a particular visit can be very much the same for twenty days or so.

> The other day on rounds with Walters [visit] I came to the conclusion he was a dirty young man. We are on female medicine, and with each patient he says, "How's the cardiac situation?" Then he goes on to listen to the heart and do a thorough chest examination. He does that every day. I thought he was getting some kicks that way. I asked an intern if it wasn't unusual to do chest exams on every female patient. He answered, "Walters is in the heart station, and this is his specialty." A student who was standing nearby asked me if I had made rounds with Tower last month, then asked how many times Tower mentioned a specific medical problem. I had counted at least a dozen times in one day. The student said, "That's his specialty, and he stays with it day after day, so it gets to be a lot of the same each day. Walters is a chest man, so for this month we see a lot of what interests him day after day." [July 4, 1964]

Interns think that because they select the patients they have control over what will be discussed. Many times I heard, "You maneuver a visit to a problem that interests you and let him talk it up." In fact, visits resist such maneuvers by refusing to talk about problems outside their specialties.

> When the visit asked for a diagnosis, the intern said, "My diagnosis is leukemia and urinary tract infection, but I'm waiting for the results of some lab work before making a definitive diagnosis." The visit [Manners] asked, "What do you think is the important problem?" The intern, Reed, said, "We would like to prove a diagnosis of malabsorption." Manners nodded. The assistant resident [Madge] asked, "What is it?" Manners looked around the table. He was on the edge of his chair. He asked Madge, "Why don't you tell him?" Madge gave some explanation. Landfeld asked, "How come you don't hear about

it?" Manners said, "It's not that well-defined a disease, because there are not many cases. It's also something I don't know a great deal about, and I would like to get off the subject."

Landfeld asked, "Is it new?" Manners said it had been around for at least 15 years. Madge asked a question about anemia and Manners said, "You've got me. I don't know a thing about it and have had no personal experience with it whatsoever. I would rather talk about something else. Let's see what we have on the ward." On our way to the ward, Landfeld said to me, "He's an endocrinologist. You can tell he's not a hematologist." [October 21, 1964]

This incident is typical. The specialty of a particular visit determines the content of his teaching. No matter how they try, residents and interns cannot maneuver the visit as they say they can. The price they must pay for the teaching they receive is to accept the visit's definition of what is and what is not for him to teach. An attempt to change the content of his teaching is easily resisted. The visit simply invokes the rule that the group will talk about something he knows about. Interns thus pay further for their teaching by limiting their inquiries to the interests of whoever is visiting at the time.

Though the interns are not entirely satisfied with this limitation, it is precisely what makes the relationship rewarding for the visiting physician, who considers visiting rounds primarily to be for their benefit. The experience is profitable, they say, because it gives them a chance to bring themselves up to date by discussing the problems of their particular specialties with interns and students.

Interns, on the other hand, play the game because the contact allows them to claim specialized assistance with particularly difficult problems. Interns can, when they need to, present the visit with a difficult problem about which he does know something. They can also use him as a consultant. A claim for assistance of this sort is different from the claim they make for teaching.

White, a student, had presented a 36-year-old patient. "While you're here, there is something I would like to ask you," Powers [intern] said to Schwartz [visit]. He had a patient's chart in his hand and asked Schwartz to look at an electro-cardiogram. Powers asked, "Would you call this a normal electrocardiogram?" Schwartz looked, then said, "Of course I would; I have." Pointing to the top of the EKG he said, "That's my name." He had signed as the physician who interpreted it. Powers laughed and said, "How about that? It's embarrassing. But could you explain why you thought it was normal?" The visit did. I knew that Powers knew Schwartz had read the EKG. When I asked why he did what he did, Powers said, "I knew why he called it normal; but he was here, and I had the chance to have him explain it to me, I probably would never have had an explanation if he wasn't here." [August 21, 1964]

The relationship with the visiting physician, then, is one of social exchange. Interns limit their interests in exchange for instruction. Because they benefit, they reciprocate by setting the stage for visiting physicians. The visit, in turn, gets satisfaction from teaching and earns the regard of interns. Further, interns get help with particular problems while the specialist gets to see more cases related to his work. Thus the relationship benefits both participants, though the benefits are less than both participants would like them to be.

THE CONSULTING PHYSICIANS

A visiting physician uses the patients presented to him only to illustrate the universal, rather than to deal with particular aspects of a given case. From him the interns learn generalizations about diseases and their etiology, progression, and management. But interns have to handle the immediate problems of specific patients. For this they need teaching less than advice and assistance in the management of disease as they encounter it on the wards. They get that sort of information from consulting physicians.

Many physicians at Boston City Hospital are established authorities in the various medical specialties. Others are competent younger men who are completing residencies or conducting research under the direction of established physicians. These are the residents, fellows, and clinical investigators who work in the research divisions of the Thorndike Laboratory or in the hospital's departments and specialty clinics. Each such group is organized around some special skill or area of knowledge and takes a special interest in a particular kind of patient. Like the visiting physicians, these men are interested in the universal aspects of medical problems. They are not concerned with routine patient care. But they make ward rounds regularly and give advice or assistance with particular aspects of specific patients' problems. They are the consulting physicians.

Though a visiting physician may occasionally serve as a consultant, physicians representing each of the research divisions, departments, or clinics regularly offer this service. There are arrangements by which interns may get immediate consultations or request regular ones. Each group of specialists usually has someone on call at all times. When an emergency consultation is requested, consultants usually come to the ward immediately. If there is no emergency, however, interns must follow a standard procedure of submitting a written request for advice or assistance. The request may be delivered to a particular consultant or passed on to the night float, who distributes all such requests. Since the night float does not distribute the requests until the morning after he receives them, there is some advantage to personal delivery. When a physician receives a request for consultation, he is expected to see the patient concerned as soon as possible. Interns would like to have a consultation the day after they request it. If they follow the established procedure, they should have no difficulty getting it.

But interns do not get help by simply asking for it, though the only formal condition for a consultation is a need for advice and assistance. Interns supposedly need not meet any other conditions or incur any obligations. In fact, though, their relationship with consulting physicians is not unconditional. There is an exchange involved.

The major condition of this exchange is the same as that with visiting physicians. That is, interns must seek help only with problems relevant to the experience, knowledge, and interests of the consultant. Otherwise, they can run into trouble.

"In the staff dining room I sat next to Brook [consulting physician]. "Well, will you be available to see a patient today?" Samuels [intern] asked. Brook said, "No, I have the weekend off. I'm going to take a long weekend. I will be here late Monday. Why don't you put in for a consult?" Samuels asked, "You are at the Heart Station?" Brook nodded and said, "Yes, just write out a consult request and drop it in my box." "We usually leave it for the night float," Samuels said, "and I wrote one a week ago." Brook asked if Samuels had requested him specifically, or if he had just requested a consult. "I asked for you specifically," Samuels replied. "It's strange that I haven't received it," Brook said, "but it may be in my box now. I haven't been over to the station today." Samuels told Brook that he had clinics on Wednesday and missed Brook at the rounds he made with his group on the wards. "Well," said Brook, "I'll be there Monday and I'll stop in. How would that be?" Samuels said, "That would be great. I'll expect you then on the ward."

Brook got up and left the table. Almost immediately Stern [intern] said, "If you're having trouble getting consults, you should write out a list of questions that'll grab him. You shouldn't just request a consult. I think some questions that would interest him would get him on the ward." Samuels said, "I'm not having trouble getting consults, but I guess this one could have gone better and I would have had it sooner." Samuels was obviously, in my opinion, having trouble getting consults. [July 3, 1964]

When a consulting physician is requested to advise an intern on a problem that doesn't especially interest him, he takes his time responding, if he answers at all. The intern must, therefore, always try to capture his interest. This endeavor often inspires interns to amazing literary efforts when writing a request for a consultation. They try to convey to the consultant that they have thought about the case and have some important questions. If this fails, they resort to other plans.

We went to see a patient on the wards with Peterson, the visiting physician, who asked Davis, an intern, about the patient's stool. "I have not," said Davis, "been able to coax the GI [gastrointestinal] group to look at her stool. I've looked at it, but I can't really tell a thing." Peterson asked, "The GI group aren't interested in her?" "You can say that, but I can't," said Davis. The other interns laughed. Peterson nodded and said, "I know it's hard to get them moving." Davis told Peterson that he thought he had interested the X-ray group in the patient. "I've contacted them and they're trying to work her in some time." Peterson said that this was OK but that he thought Davis should also get the GI group interested. "I'm telling them both that the other is interested. If a free-enterprise system works, I should get some results. If I can get a little competition going between them, I may get both groups to help." There was more laughter. [October 21, 1964]

The consulting physicians have other duties. They make rounds of patients with other members of their group. Most of them also spend time doing laboratory work. All the patients the interns want them to see may not interest them since their problems may not bear on current research or add to their knowledge of disease. Interns recognize the implications of these circumstances for their relationship with consulting physicians.

"Most of the consults aren't too good," Taylor [intern] told me. "They don't have the time to sit down and talk over all your patients with you. They are not interested in all your patients. You could get a lot more out of them if they had more time. The nerve consults are probably the best because they have more time. They do full-time consulting."

I asked, "Is it easy to get a consult?" Taylor said, "No. Well, if you really need them, yes. But from day to day, no. Most of them are more interested in doing research. They begrudge you the time and try to make consulting the least of their activity. If you have a difficult problem or any unusual one, they come. You don't use them just for advice. You usually put in for a consult because you want procedures done that only one of the group can do. You usually go to your own house staff for advice because they have as much to say and are actually better than many of the consults. The assistant resident and the senior resident can usually answer most of your questions. And if you have an esoteric question you can ask the consults who are probably working on it." [April 19, 1965]

The practice of seeking advice from residents is a result of the limits consultants set on their relationships with interns. Implicit in the practice is the intern's recognition of the conditions that justify a request for a consultation. First, the request must concern problems that interest the consulting physician. The physician whose advice is sought does, of course, benefit by this recognition of his superior knowledge, but he must pay with his time. Since he has a superordinate position to begin with, he may not consider the reward worth the price. Interns must, therefore, present their requests as opportunities for consultants to see interesting patients. Finally, they must not seek consultation unless their questions cannot be answered by residents on the wards. Consultants do not add to their reputations by answering questions that can be answered by people with less experience and training. And they do not add to their experience or knowledge by seeing patients with routine problems. Interns are aware of the terms of their relationships with consultants.

> Pere [intern] said, "Well, the consult should be available at all times when the intern wants to see him. Whenever the intern feels the need for information about the diagnosis and treatment of specific diseases, the consult should provide the information freely. He should help the intern decide what to do, but never take the situation out of the intern's hands." He laughed, and I asked, "What?"
>
> "Well," Pere said, "believe me, consults can be obnoxious. I don't know why some of them behave as they do but they are not willing to part with information freely. I don't know why, but some consults make you feel sorry you asked them to come see a patient. They seem to be busy with other things. The kind of information you want isn't the kind you always get. You want to know as much as they can tell you about a patient's disease and the possible diagnoses or ways of treating the patient. They come on the ward and talk with you. Maybe they give you a reference or two, but they don't tell you everything they know about a disease. The consults act like they're sacred bearers of the word when you ask for the kind of information you really want. You do better talking

most of your patients over with the residents. But if it's a disease the consult is really interested in, he tells you a lot. A lot you didn't even ask for. You call in a hematology consult, for example, and he says it's probably this but it could also be that. He tells you to do this test to rule one or the other problem out and tells you to treat the patient with this or that. That's routine. When the patient interests him or you have some real questions, he tells you he just happens to be doing a study on this and could he perform a test on your patient, or would you watch the patient carefully. Then he tells you what he knows and what is being done and what the data is and so on. This helps me because he gives me more than I asked for. He also gets me involved in something that relates to his interest and my patient." [December 23, 1964]

Generally, interns accept the limitations placed on their relationship with consulting physicians. This does not mean, however, that they are satisfied with that relationship. They are displeased because consultations are often difficult to obtain and because they believe that the consultant often benefits more than they do from a consultation.

I asked Daley [intern] if he was going to request a consultation. He said, "I'm at the point where I feel I can handle things pretty much by myself. When I do have an interesting problem, I like to talk it over with a consultant, but the fact of the matter is that I don't need him as much now as I did at the beginning of the year. I still put in for as many, and I still get as many as I did before. But the benefits to me and the patient are not great. If I were a consult, I think I would feel more responsibility to the interns. I would teach more. They only give you essential routine most of the time. I get the feeling that it's not for my benefit but for theirs."

I asked how the consultants benefit from a consultation. He replied, "Well, like this lady here with anemia and neurological complications. I will write a request for a neurology consult. What I am saying to him is here she is, come and see her. She's got some interesting complications. I don't need him to tell me she's sick. But she would be an interesting patient for him to see. I think half the consults I request are like that." [May 25, 1965]

There is another aspect to the situation:

> When we had finished visiting rounds the assistant resident asked, "What do you think of Tucker [consulting physician] today?" The intern, Newton, said, "He was great. He had a lot to say. You know, he can take a temperature, pulse, ask a couple of questions and suddenly he has the whole perspective. You see the patient and the problem in an entirely different way. You have a new slant on the disease and the treatment." Another intern, Markman, said, "You know one thing about Tucker, though, you have to watch him. He looks at you and says, 'Leukemia, what's leukemia?' He does it in such a way that if you don't watch it you get sucked in. Then you're giving him all the latest poop. He gets a lot more that way than you do." [July 29, 1964]

Since a consultation may not benefit an intern or his patient, interns could be expected to request them less often or not at all. A consultation, however, is not always a request for advice; it may involve assistance of another sort. If an intern is attending a handicapped patient, for example, he may request a physical therapy consultation. Later, when he is ready to discharge the patient, the fact that he had the consultation will facilitate the process. We have already seen how a consultation with a physician from the diabetes clinic saved an intern the time and trouble of cutting toenails. Consultants can often assist interns by performing special procedures.

> "Tell me," asked Fox, an intern, "can you do a bone marrow in the outpatient department?" "No," said Myer, assistant resident, "you're not set up to do it. It's not complicated to do. In fact, it's easy. But you're not set up." Laughingly Fox said, "Just give me a needle." "No," said Myer, "you don't want to do it that way. Just schedule a hematology consult next time your patient will be at the clinic. Then they will come over and do it for you. That's the way to do it. No problem for you." "Do you think we need a bone marrow?" asked Fox. "You don't need much," Myer said.
>
> Henry, a senior resident, said, "They'll just grab a hunk and smear a couple of slides. It doesn't take a big piece, and they don't mind doing it."

"OK," Fox said, "it sounds easy. I'll do it." [April 13, 1965]

Interns also continue to request consultations because they can occasionally select patients whose problems interest them as well as the consulting physicians:

> I asked, "Do you mean to say you selected that patient especially for the consult?" "Yes," Sudman replied, "I wanted to know more about endocrine disease. I had a problem I knew they were interested in so I requested a consult. I gave them a patient they could say a lot about." [January 20, 1965]

Finally, interns continue to request consultations because they are expected to do so. The consulting physicians are interested in particular kinds of patients for their own reasons, either to further their knowledge or to advance their research. Whatever they need patients for, it is almost impossible for them to keep watch for the kinds they need. Interns do this for them.

> "Think of it this way," said Hoyt [intern], "as a big box. All the patients are in a box. The Thorndike people have to know what's in the box. The patients can't run away. The Thorndike people make rounds. But they may miss a patient they really want to see. You keep an eye out for the patients they want, the patients they need to do their research. If you find one, you give them a call." [January 20, 1965]

Interns are repeatedly told that clinical investigation is a part of the best medicine. "The conferences are all quite good," they are told, "but the best teaching occurs where there is clinical investigation." The Thorndike physicians tell interns that the physicians on the wards are an important part of the Harvard Medical Unit. What that part is they learn from the clinical investigators.

> We attended a conference with physicians from a specialty group. "The Thorndike people are here to help with diagnosis and treatment," Dr. Newpril told us. "As the year goes on you will need our help less, but we will still depend a great deal on you to pick out the problems we're interested in. I can't emphasize too much our dependence on you. What we can do for you is not that easy to answer, but we will always be

available as you need us. We will also try to keep you informed of what we need. Any patient with complications, abnormalities, certainly deserves our attention. Though it is common that many patients with, for example, diabetes have other abnormalities, we will like to see all such patients and would be very appreciative if you would give us a call. We rely on you to get the material for us." [August 4, 1964]

Interns obligate themselves to consulting physicians the first time they seek their help. In exchange for valuable information or services they must furnish the consultants with information about patients who might be useful in clinical investigations. Though interns may not need much advice after they have been at the hospital for a time, they obligate themselves during the first few months of the internship, and they are expected to discharge that debt for the rest of the year. In time, though, they themselves begin to set conditions for further service to consultants.

> Seaman [intern] told me that he has become a ward politician. I said that a Thorndike physician had told me he had to be a politician too, that he had to get along with the interns. "Oh sure," said Seaman, "the reason they have to get along with us is because they want our patients to do experiments on and that sort of thing. If we don't care for what they are doing, then we are not going to tell them about patients we have, or say you can do what you want with my patient. Since the intern really has the say about what's going to be done with his patient, unless he gets some kind of benefit from the consultants, he's not going to let them do what they want. Why should I say, 'Sure, do a bone-marrow biopsy on this patient'? I think, in order for them to have the privilege of doing things with my patients, they have to offer some services too. I make them tell me everything they are going to do, and I want it explained to me." [April 19, 1965]

When interns keep clinical investigators informed and permit them to use their patients, they obligate those physicians to provide more than information regarding essential routine. By discharging their obligations, interns place themselves in a position to demand teaching performance from consulting physicians.

The threat that they will do so is always a possibility, though I did not once see an intern refuse clinical investigators the permission to use his patients. An intern occasionally complained that the clinical investigators were using his patients as guinea pigs, but he knew that his complaint would not influence those in authority. Interns are, in fact, told that they may not always understand why certain procedures are necessary, or that they may think these things are not in the best interests of their patients. When they have such doubts, they are supposed to consult the clinical investigator. They do not need to be told that any difference of opinion will be resolved in favor of the latter. It is, therefore, more the threat than the actual exercise of sanctions by interns that places them in a position to negotiate for teaching performances.

One final fact suggests that the relationship between interns and consultants is social exchange. Interns have the least difficulty in obtaining consultations with Thorndike physicians. When they request help from physicians affiliated with other medical schools than Harvard, they are often told that those physicians are very busy, and they must wait. Generally, a Thorndike physician will, if all conditions are met, provide consultation as soon as possible. Interns think that this difference results from loyalty to the Harvard Medical Services. That may be so, but there is another explanation: Interns are in a better position to negotiate with Harvard physicians than with those from other medical schools. The Thorndike physicians recognize their obligation to interns who are supplying patients for clinical investigations. They get valuable information from interns and reciprocate by furnishing consultation when the occasion arises. Physicians on the services of other medical schools do not obtain many patients this way and therefore may not feel indebted to the Harvard interns. In other words, the conditions for social exchange do not always exist between Harvard interns and non-Harvard physicians.

EXCHANGE WITH SUBORDINATES

Interns must establish and maintain relationship with nursing and ancillary personnel. They need the services of a variety of people if they are to get their own work done. For example, an intern decides what the patient's bed, board, and general care will be, but the nurse is the one who implements the decisions. Interns also decide what tests should be made, but the nurses collect necessary specimens and the technicians do the tests. Interns need the cooperation of the people who provide such services.

The medical degree empowers interns to order the services of nurses, aides, orderlies, and technicians. The hospital delegates to them the responsibility for patients and gives them the power to coordinate the patient-care activities of subordinates. An intern is supposed to be able to tell other people what to do. So long as he observes hospital policy, he can command nurses to carry out his orders, porters to transport patients, and technicians to do laboratory tests. By exercising the power they have, interns should be able to obtain the services they need.

Interns do not, however, exercise their power. A number of circumstances make it difficult for them to do so. Because there is a shortage of all kinds of personnel at Boston City Hospital, an intern who indiscriminately commanded services would be taking an advantage that might earn him the disapproval of other interns. To demand all he needs of limited services deprives other interns who are also in need.

Besides obliging interns to be judicious in their exercise of power, the shortage of personnel also increases the value of services. There is a great demand for services and too few people to supply it. Since interns value the services but do not in fact command them, the conditions for social exchange obtain. Interns must induce service personnel to help them by offering them something in exchange. Since they are dependent on subordinates, their power over them is reduced.

Other forces operate to reduce the power of interns. For one thing, as we have seen, they rely on subordinates to teach them the ropes. For another, a subordinate might possibly refuse to obey an order. The intern would have to respond by making threats which would be pointless unless he would carry them out. Residents tell interns this is impossible, because employees are political appointees and have the support of administrators.

Interns assume that hospital administrators will resolve any difficulty in favor of employees because administrators depend for their jobs on the good will of politicians. They may well be inclined to favor employees over interns. Whether or not they do is less important than the interns' belief that they do, from which they conclude that they have little if any actual power.

If interns had power over subordinates, subordinates would be anxious to serve them in order to earn their good will. But since they do not actually have such power, subordinates are not much concerned with pleasing them. They may even have to be reminded that they are obliged to follow orders. Unable to command, interns must bargain for cooperation. Since their relationships with their subordinates are not really between people of unequal power, these relationships are social exchanges.

The means by which interns obligate subordinates to serve them is the crux of their relationship. An intern who tolerates unimportant omissions and delays gains an advantage over subordinates. He earns a reputation for being tolerant and obligates subordinates to please him because he is reasonable. A tolerant attitude also asserts the intern's right to service by reminding subordinates that they owe him more than he is asking.

> The patient had been complaining about the amount of medication he had to take. A nurse asked Grant [intern] to have a talk with him. The patient got out of bed and started to walk down the corridor. "If you're going to void," Grant told him, "don't forget to take that jar with you. You have to save it in a jar." The patient shrugged and came back to the bed to pick up the jar. After the patient left, Grant turned to me and said, "As far as I know, he needs everything he is getting. I may have to rewrite my orders but it looks right to me."
>
> A patient in another bed called Grant, saying: "Doctor, you said you would take this out. Please take this [intravenous] needle out." Grant walked over to the patient. A nurse who was in the room said, "I'll get it for you. I'll do it." Grant

started to take the needle out, but the nurse came over and said, "I said I would do it for you. You don't have to do it." Smiling, Grant said: "You're right, I don't. I didn't hear you. I know you have a lot to do, but if I heard you I would let you do it. You can finish, if you want." We walked away from the bed.

"I didn't hear her," said Grant. "I'm always willing to let the nurse do anything she wants. The nurse is always right. Never disagree with the nurse. I don't ask them to do too much, and I never disagree with them. That's the way to do it." I asked him why. He said, "If they're right this time, they'll just be a little more willing to do what I want them to do next time. So, as far as I'm concerned, they are always right. They'll do anything for me." I laughed and asked: "Is that the secret of your success?" "Yes," Grant said, "a good intern knows more than how to care for his patients. He knows how to get things done, and that means getting along with people." [September 30, 1964]

Merely agreeing with people is not enough. Genuine tolerance requires the interns to do some things for themselves.

We were making work rounds. Little [intern] walked into the patient cubicle. "What are we looking for?' Boyd [intern] asked. Little said, "We want to clear up her lungs." Boyd asked, "Do you think we will be able to clear them up here, in the hospital? What are we doing to clear up her lungs?" Little told him that he had not been able to identify anything by sputum sample. He was just positioning the patient to help clear the lungs. The assistant resident explained that position was very important in these cases. "If she just lies there, she won't clear up," he said. "You should order her turned every 30 minutes." Boyd said, "That would really require more nursing than we have available. You'll have to do it yourself." With Boyd's help, Little got the patient out of bed. [July 31, 1964]

"You know," Cohen said, "a lot of my time is spent on things that are not directly related to patient care." "Like what?" I asked. "Well, like having to do a drainage. You have to do it yourself. Things that I have to do like that would be done by technicians at other hospitals. The technicians would probably do the physical therapy, coughs, breathing exercises, things like that. I think many of these things have very little to do with being a doctor and are more things paramedical personnel should do. But in this hospital, there are not enough paramedical people, so we do these things ourselves." [May 3, 1965]

Tolerance also requires interns to spend their time running around the hospital. The following excerpt from my notes again illustrates running around, which is so much a part of the intern's job, and the tolerance of the conditions which require him to do so.

> Yost and I were having coffee. He had just returned after picking up some blood. "You have to be organized," he said. "You learn it during the internship. Another thing you have to learn is to keep good personal relations with the nurses and so on. This hospital is like a little ward, you know. You have to be willing to do a lot. Like I knew I could have this blood I needed if I went over and got it myself. People would be too busy to deliver it. You have to run around to keep things going well. They are overworked, and you have to keep them happy."
> "Do you work at keeping people happy?"
> "Oh boy!" he said, "You have to! You manipulate for all you're worth. If you send down an X-ray and don't go over, you may not get it. So you go over. They still may tell you they're all booked up. But you can say, 'Come on, I'm a good guy.' 'OK,' they say, 'just this once.' It's true for lab technicians, everyone here. Just because you're a doctor is no guarantee your patients are going to get what they need. Man, you've got to go and get it for them." [April 19, 1965]

When they go to get what they need, interns must be tolerant. They cannot rush the people who are serving them. The point here is that going in person is not doing things the way they should be done. Subordinates feel that requests made in person are special; they do not feel obliged to grant special requests. A request made as it should be, usually in writing, must be granted in due time. But special requests disrupt the routine and subordinates reserve the right to refuse. When he grants a special request, however, a subordinate does more than he has to and thus obliges interns to continue being tolerant.

> Since Boyd wanted some X-rays, we went over to get them. They had not been developed and were in a pile on the table. He picked his pictures out of the pile. A clerk, who hadn't offered to help us look for them, asked, "You sure you have the right ones?" "I took the one that had my ticket on it," Boyd said, "and the one under it, right?" The technician said that was right. "Is there a chance of having them developed?" asked Boyd. "Why won't you go talk to the man?" said the clerk. "If he isn't too busy, he could do it for you now." We went to the developing room. There were some people standing around talking, and we had to wait until they left. Boyd asked if the pictures could be developed. The technician said, "Maybe, if you don't make this a habit." He stepped into the darkroom. When he came out, Boyd asked how long it would take. "Don't know," said the technician, "five or six minutes. Why, can't you wait?" "Yes," said Boyd, "if it'll only take a few minutes, we'll wait." I said, "We can come back later." Boyd laughed. "If we do that," he said, "we'll never see those pictures again. He'll do it for me now, but he wants me to know it's a favor. But then that's the way it is at this hospital. You scratch their backs, and they scratch yours." [April 7, 1965]

Thus, there are the conditions of social exchange between interns and hospital employees. If subordinates do not repay the interns' tolerance, they violate the conditions of the relationships.

> An intern, Wright, said, "I think you have to be fair with hospital employees and they should be fair back. A lot of times they're not fair. I mean some of them are just dishonest. I want to get an X-ray taken. I write the requisition and take it down myself. You have to make sure it gets there. I don't rely on anyone else to do it for me. I set the thing up to get a chest film. A technician says he will be up to the ward to take a portable film, but he never comes. That kind of thing is dishonest." [June 2, 1965]

When interns call hospital employees dishonest, they refer to violations of the conditions of their relationship, not to illegal activity of any sort. Since interns have little or no recourse, they can only hope that violations are the exceptions that prove the rules of social exchange. Thus, they are more dependent on and committed to exchange relationships than are subordinates.

Besides being tolerant, interns do have some other ways of inducing subordinates to cooperate with them. Though their power is limited, they have at least as much status as any other group at the hospital. This is capital, which interns can expend as they need to. The medical degree, of course, is one source of interns' high stature. They are members of the most honored and lucrative of professions. In addition, their social origins are middle class. Nursing is not an established profession, and most nurses at the hospital are only striving to be middle class. Other employees have even less status than nurses. Thus interns are socially superior to virtually all the people with whom they must work.

"The fact that many people find it rewarding to associate with superiors means that those of superior status can furnish rewards, and expect a return for them, merely by associating with others of lower status." If this is so, it is not surprising that most hospital personnel find it rewarding to associate with doctors. This means that interns, who have the status of physicians, can furnish rewards for which they may expect a return from the people with whom they must work. Interns have little to lose by associating with subordinates. They cannot lose power, because they have little. Treating subordinates as equals can only ease the relationships by removing an impediment to sociability. The reduction of social differences between them can only further obligate subordinates.

> The senior resident had called a meeting of the interns and assistant residents. I was with Peters [assistant resident]. "Maybe we should ask our sociologist [pointing to me] to tell us something about my next topic," said the senior resident. I told him I would have a lot to say later, but not now. He laughed. "I'd like to suggest," he continued, "that you interns make an effort to talk with the nurses every chance you get. I think some nurses are put off by what they think are social differences. They feel that they are the social inferiors of the

medical staff. Not the professional inferiors, but the social inferiors. They don't quite feel equal to you. I think you have to make an effort to overcome this. One way I think that you can do this is by sitting down with nurses for a cup of coffee. There are other things you can do but I think the time between 10 and 10:30 A.M. can be used for coffee and cake and talk. I think this is part of your job."

"I agree," said Peters. "It's important to talk with the nurses. There's one thing, for example, that I don't think is very well known, and that's that the final route for all medications and drugs is on the white cards that nurses carry. You can write orders and make notes until you're blue in the face, but if it's not on their white cards, it will never be delivered. When you are sitting with the nurses, it's a good idea to take a look at those cards to make sure everything is on them that you want on them. You'll really get your work done if you do this."

"That's right," said the senior resident. "If you ask the girls to bring in coffee and cake, they'll be more than happy to do so. In any case," he concluded, "the thing is to remember to get along with the nurses." [June 29, 1965]

To get the nurses' cooperation interns must establish egalitarian relationships. The coffee break is an important overture interns make to overcome the impediments to a sociable and profitable relationship with nurses. They make an effort to spend this time with nurses though there are many other things they could do with a free half-hour. The results of these interludes are usually what interns hope they will be.

I was waiting for Dewey and Cook [interns] to come up, but today, unusual as it was, they did not come up to the third-floor laboratory. It was after 10, so I decided to go down to the ward and see what was up. I found Dewey preparing medications, a good reason for staying on the ward, but not in the kitchen. Cook was also in the kitchen, writing in charts and the order book. The nurse who had been on the ward left yesterday to have a baby. Today there were two new nurses. I sat down next to Cook, who said, "Happy to report it's a great morning!" He returned to the charts and order book. "Hey," he said, "this patient has gone home! How come the sheet is still in the book?" One nurse said, "We figure if we leave it, you'll write some orders by accident that we won't have to do." Both nurses giggled. Cook smiled and continued to write orders. A nurse asked me if I wanted a cup of coffee. "No," I said, "but it's the first time I've been offered a cup in the morning." The other nurse said, "It'll give us a chance to get our notes straight." Cook said that it was a good idea, and Dewey nodded his head. It was a rather pleasant get-together, relaxed with a give-and-take. This was the first time [approximately two weeks had passed] that I saw any people except the old nurse and aides seated in the kitchen.

Cook asked the nurse if there was an eye clinic at the hospital. "Yes," she said, "but why?" "I have a patient," Cook replied, "that wants to be fitted for glasses." The nurse said, "It's best to let her handle it through the clinic, and not on the ward. They don't like to do it on the ward." "Should I," asked Cook, "handle it at the outpatient department?" The nurse nodded. [July 8, 1964]

By making such overtures to nurses interns expend some status, but in return they gain the nurses' good will. Nurses appreciate the time interns take to have coffee with them. In fact, they point out to interns the benefits of doing so. When the nurse remarked that coffee breaks offered a good way of keeping the work straight, she was urging them to continue the relationship they started. Her accepting the role of teaching Cook the ropes was also reciprocity, a further inducement to continue the exchange relationship.

Interns do, however, have to make some greater expenditures of status. The difference between their stature and the nurses' is not so great as that between interns and other hospital personnel. In dealing with clerks or technicians, for example, interns must yield a great deal of status, since these people are not even quasiprofessional.

Warren [intern] picked up a telephone and, looking at a card he had taken from his pocket, dialed a number. When he got his party, he said, "I wonder if you would be very kind and give me something very important off a record you have. I need to know where a patient was transferred from. Could you look it up for me?" I said, "He is being very polite." Smith [assistant resident] said, "That's what I told him to be. I told him to play up to the girls in the record room so he won't have any trouble getting what he wants. He's learning." [June 29, 1965]

To get things done, interns must reduce the social difference that separates them from their subordinates. They do so by deferring to hospital employees just as they would to people with equal or higher status. Like the coffee break, deference is an overture acknowledging interns' dependence on subordinates. It implies that their relationship is not one of unequal power but of egalitarian exchange. Interns usually define their tolerance and courtesy toward subordinates as "diplomacy." When they become impatient with employees, they know they are violating the conditions of their relationship.

> Boren [intern] told me that the patient who had been saved by resuscitation the day before had died. "Did you hear what happened?" he asked, then explained that they wanted to take the cadaver away and change the sheets, but that other patients refused to pull their drapes shut. The attendant who had come for the cadaver pulled the drapes shut around him and waited and waited, but the patients just walked around. The cadaver could not be taken away with patients walking around. The intern had finally shouted: "Nurse, get the patients in bed and pull those drapes so we can pull this cadaver the hell out of here!" "How about that?" Boren asked. "Is that being diplomatic, or is that being diplomatic? I know," he said, "it's not the way to do it, but it had to be done." [July 1, 1964]

Interns are usually extremely tolerant and very polite. "Well, you know best," they acquiesce, implying that their relationship is one between equals. Interns could, of course, be intolerant, but they realize that intolerance would not obtain the assistance and services they need.

> Grant [intern] came on the ward and announced that the biochemistries were back. He handed a stack of sheets to Newton [intern], one for each patient for whom tests had been requested. Newton looked the sheets over and asked, "Aren't the ones I sent in yesterday back yet? I'll have a fit.

How about the X-rays? Are they back yet?" "No," said Grant, "they're not, and having a fit won't do any good." Newton laughed and said, "I guess you have to be diplomatic." [June 29, 1964]

In an attempt to get things done without subverting an egalitarian relationship, many interns adopt a kidding approach to the people with whom they must work.

> We were in the lab. Smith [intern] was at a desk writing in charts. I said, "I thought you would be home in bed by now." "I'll have you know," said Smith, "I'm the Dr. Kildare of BCH, and if I don't do my work, Dr. Gillespie [nodding toward the assistant resident] will chew my ass out." The assistant resident told me that Smith did nothing but bitch. "If the work was in trouble," retorted Smith, "an AR would be the one who screwed things up. And an intern would get his ass and the work out of trouble." "If he worked as much as he talks, we could all go home," said the assistant resident. Laughter.
> Newton [intern] said to me: "That Smith, he's a funny man. You know, he looks like he doesn't care, but he gets his work done. I don't know how. He's not diplomatic, but he gets his work done. He's funny." "Funny how?" "Ha-ha funny," said Newton. "He goes around bitching and complaining. He tells people straight out what's on his mind. The nurses don't particularly like him, but he doesn't take a thing from them. That's what I mean. He can kid with people, but he puts them down too. A lot of times people don't know if he's kidding or not. It's effective." I asked, "How's it effective?" "I guess . . ." Newton said, "I mean it works for him. He gets people to do what he wants them to that way, though it wouldn't work for the rest of us." [January 6, 1965]

The kidding approach to subordinates does not always work. Smith, for example, got along with some people:

> Smith had a blood chemistry he wanted done, so he took it down himself. When he entered the lab, he immediately asked in a song, "Who's going to do a blood chemistry? Who's going to do a blood chemistry? Which pretty girl is going to do a blood chemistry for me?" The first girl he came to looked up,

smiled, and sang, "Not me. Not me." Laughing, Smith just handed her the specimen and said, "Take good care of that. That's blood, though you may not know it." [July 21, 1964]

But others did not appreciate his approach:

Smith needed some help with a patient. He looked at one of the nurses and said, "I suppose you want to go out with me." "I think you're cute," said the nurse, "but not that cute." She walked away. He turned to the other nurse and asked, "How about you?" "I don't think you're cute at all," she said, "so forget it." "How about that?" asked Smith. [June 21, 1965]

Interns compensate for their lack of actual power by inducing people to assist them. The diplomatic approach to subordinates is the most profitable way for interns to get their help. The resulting egalitarian relationship benefits subordinates by permitting them to retain control of their work. They therefore reciprocate by giving interns the service they want and need.

FAIR EXCHANGE BETWEEN INTERNS AND RESIDENTS

"The patient is my responsibility," interns say, "and the ward is the responsibility of the assistant resident." Assistant residents agree. This understanding of areas of responsibility prescribes the relationship between interns and assistant residents. The assistant resident enforces the rules established by hospital administrators and the physicians of the Harvard Medical Unit. Interns must obey those rules. The assistant residents have enough power over interns to tell them what to do. In principle the relationship is one between superior and subordinate.

In practice, though, power is not the basis of the relationship. The relationship cannot actually be prescribed, because the limits of responsibility are not obvious. When, for example, are assistant resident's instructions concerning patients a ward matter, and when are they a matter of patient care? If an assistant resident insisted that his orders be obeyed, he could be denying an intern his right to responsibility for his patients. The line between ward policy and patient care is not well defined enough

to permit interns and residents to operate according to the principle of ward organization. They must, therefore, negotiate a
relationship.

It is not the inequality of power that allows residents to
enforce rules against interns, but the great inequality of information. The assistant resident has successfully passed through
medical and other situations the intern has yet to meet and
manage. He knows how things must be done at the hospital if
they are to be done at all. Interns need to know what residents
know. They depend upon residents for advice as well as assistance and services. The intern accepts a subordinate position
because of this dependence, not because of the resident's inherent power.

> Prentice [assistant resident] and I entered the laboratory. Kauf-
> mann [intern] was waiting for us. "Can I go ahead and give
> Mr. Jones something for his pain?" He asked. "I don't see
> why not," Prentice said, "but what do you have in mind?"
> Kaufmann said he thought he would start the patient on
> demarol. Prentice thought for a minute and said, "I don't
> know, that's a little strong. There are so many things that
> will kill pain but are not strong. I think you should think
> about other medications." "What would you suggest?" asked
> Kaufmann. Prentice proposed codein. Kaufmann nodded and
> said: "I haven't fed Mr. Smith because I'm scheduling him
> for some X-rays." "Why for X-rays?" asked Prentice. "Because
> there's a block there," explained Kaufmann, "and I don't know
> where." "Why don't you do a rectal first?" asked Prentice, add-
> ing that Mr. Smith might just be impacted and a rectal
> examination would clear up the block. Kaufmann thanked
> Prentice and left to see his patients. [June 29, 1965]

> A patient was shouting. He was having leg cramps and was in
> extreme pain. "I don't know what to do," said Harris [intern].
> "I've never seen cramps like this before. What do I do?"
> "I think you give him quinine," said Booth [assistant resident].
> Harris ran to the nurses' station and returned with a book
> of drugs by name and type. He thumbed through the book
> and said: "All I can find is that it's contraindicated for renal
> disease." A student was telling another intern that these
> cramps are very painful and that something had to be done

for them. "Here it is," said Booth, who had taken the book from Harris. "It says one or two tablets. Why don't you start him on one. OK?" Harris nodded and went to get the quinine. The assistant resident and a student went over to massage the patient's legs. [July 17, 1964]

Interns have responsibility for the care of patients, but they don't always know what to do for them. They depend upon the assistant resident for advice, which they follow since they have no satisfactory alternatives. Because interns realize their inexperience, the resident can influence them without imposing his will. It is, in fact, inexperience and ignorance of the hospital which makes possible social exchange. If interns were knowledgable and experienced they would not need to comply in exchange for assistance with their work. The resident could, of course, issue orders, but advice works better, getting the same results without subverting the interns' responsibility. His advice benefits interns and places them in his debt as an exercise of power would not. The subtlety of the assistant residents' influence is not lost on interns.

Landfeld, Hertman [interns], and I were standing at the bottom of the stairs in the Peabody Building. I asked Landfeld how he felt about Goldson, his new assistant resident. He said: "I'm getting a lot out of him; he's an interesting guy. He's not after you all the time to get your work done like the other residents are." "I thought you liked your other residents," I said. "Yes," he explained, "I did. They were OK, but they have to be compulsive. Look at Booth. I don't know a more paternalistic person, but he's sneaky. He'd say 'Well, now I think we'll have to do that sometime tomorrow afternoon between 3 and 5.' That means we'll do it at four. That's how he was. It looked like he went all around the bush, but he was right on top of things. You were doing what he wanted without being told to do it. Goldson isn't as compulsive as the other assistant residents. It doesn't bother him if you let some things go. He doesn't even try to get you to do everything. He's not a scut man like the others, like all of us who have been trained here at Boston City Hospital." [April 4, 1965]

Interns do not resent the residents' advice, though they know it is how they coordinate patient care. They appreciate all the help they can get from residents.

> "The real thing is responsibility," Hertman told me. "That's what's important. Taking care of patients and making decisions, that's responsibility. But what's good about responsibility here is that you're not left on your own. The assistant resident is always around. He's not butting in, but he's there, and you can call on him if you need him. He's willing to help, but he's not telling you what to do. That's what's good about this internship." [December 2, 1964]

Interns respect the judgment of assistant residents and therefore follow their advice. The obligation they incur thereby impels them to reciprocate by complying with assistant residents' requests. There is also the threat that if they do not try to please, advice will not be forthcoming when they need it. Though the interns' dependence on them assures that their advice will be followed, residents take steps further to obligate interns.

Residents carry the hallmark of a physician. They have responsibility, and they have clinical experience, both of which the intern covets. A resident is more like a practicing physician than like an intern. He can grant rewards and expect a return for them by reducing the differences in status between himself and the interns. This in itself rewards the intern, because it indicates that he is making progress toward his chosen career. If the residents accept him as an equal, he is well on his way to being a physician. The resident understands this and is willing to play.

> "You know," Booth [assistant resident] said to me, "there's more to an internship than book learning. How to get an X-ray is an example of something that's not in the book." I nodded but said nothing. Goldson [assistant resident] asked if I had anything to say about the differences between interns, assistant residents, and senior residents. I told him I thought that residents made a conscious effort to be close to interns. "Yes," said Booth, "what would you, as a sociologist, call

that?" Laughing, I said, "A manifest effort to reduce role distance."

Smiling, Booth said, "You know, at the Massachusetts General they make no real distinction between the intern and the resident. The interns and the resident alternate on nights, and they do the same kind of work. Everything goes very well over there." "Maybe," said Goldson, "there's a point where you reduce role distance too much." Laughter. "No," said Booth, "I was a student over there, and everything was fine. The resident was still listened to." 'Man," asked Goldson, "what is this role distance?" I laughed. "I don't know," said Booth, "but treating interns as equals is important." [August 5, 1964]

The assistant residents establish an egalitarian relationship with interns by not exercising the power they have and by taking an active part in patient care. They do physical examinations of most patients, write suggestions for their care, and discuss each patient with the intern responsible, but they are careful to leave the final decisions to interns. Residents do not order but suggest, and this after they have done many of the same things that interns must do. They also work the same hours and take their meals with interns. Interns are grateful for this sort of relationship and anxious to retain the residents' good will. "Residents are people just like us," they say, "reasonable guys who remember what it was like to be an intern, so they want to be of help." Interns come to think of residents not as superiors but as friends. It is difficult not to follow the suggestions of friends, particularly when they have your best interests at heart and want to help you.

Because of the interns' dependence on them, residents have no trouble coordinating their efforts when the interns are newcomers. But after interns learn the ropes, the relationship will not persist as social exchange unless residents have something besides advice and friendship to offer.

"When I got here, I thought Mayer [assistant resident] was a kindred spirit. Now, I think he's a little too much." "He's on your back too much?" I asked. "No," said King, "but he was just doing too much for me. I think that a little distance

would be better for me and the patient." "Do you think," I
askd, "that you were too close to him?" "Oh no," King explained. "By distance I mean he should sit back and think
about what is going on rather than actually doing it. I remember once I was admitting somebody who wasn't too
interesting, and there was another patient, a comatose patient.
He went down and did the same kind of business I did with
the other patient. These weren't his patients." [May 25,
1965]

When interns no longer need so much advice, they resent too
much of it. At the beginning of the year they have every
reason to admit their inferiority. No one expects them to know
all they need to know, nor to be able to do all they must do.
Later in the year, when they have gained experience, they find
continued advice from residents degrading. A resident who gives
advice when interns no longer need it implicitly denies their
progress. "When they are new," assistant residents explain,
"they're asking us about everything, but later they think we're
a pain in the ass, and that we just get in the way." This is not
to say that interns do not want advice later in the year. Rather,
they want less advice and more assistance.

I asked Lynd [intern] why he had wanted this particular
internship. "The responsibility," he said. "That's why. You're
allowed to do a lot on your own." I asked him if he had the
responsibility from the start. "It really depends," he explained,
"on you and the assistant resident. You depend on him for a
lot at first. In the beginning, he's with you a lot. For two
or three days he will go to admitting with you, but after that
you should be on your own. That sheet they give you says
the AR goes with you to the admitting floor each time. He
really doesn't. He will if you really want him to, but by then
you can go on your own. But he can help a lot of times by
drawing blood or running over to get this or that. That way
he's a great help to you." [December 1, 1964]

The more experience the intern acquires, the less he values the
resident's. The logical conclusion of this decreasing dependency
might be anarchy, when the residents have nothing left to
exchange. But residents have ways to replenish the power they

have willingly depleted. They still know more medicine than the interns do, and can continue the relationship by providing service and acting as a source of information.

Experienced interns are less amenable to control and try to set their own level and direction of effort. Though they now act independently of residents, they still accept their direction when there is a question of what should be done.

> With only a few weeks left, Hertman [intern] and I had a talk. "I worked out my own way of doing things," he said, "though the assistant resident still sets the pace. It depends on how much he demands of an intern. He points out things about patients that you may let slip. I think he lets some things slip too. You may have a sneaking suspicion that a patient has some disease or other, a real long shot. The AR might think he doesn't. You can go ahead and do all the tests to find out. On the other hand, the AR may think the patient has something significantly wrong, and you don't think it is significant. You go ahead and find out. The AR, in the sense that we usually do what he says, has authority. We don't differ very much or often, but when we do it's his word, and we try to do the things he wants us to do. We usually think alike about most problems, so there's never any trouble. There isn't even trouble when he asks us to do things we don't think have to be done." [June 2, 1965]

When an intern and a resident disagree on medical procedure, they usually resolve the difference by seeking the opinion of a specialist. The consulting physician views the request as nothing more than a need for his advice on a difficult medical problem, not an attempt to settle a problem of authority. Consultation is not, therefore, a threat to the intern and residents cannot use it as a means to assert power. A resident uses consultants to demonstrate his superior knowledge of medicine, not to coerce interns.

> I was with Hedge [intern] and Goldson [assistant resident], who were examining an old women admitted to the hospital with chest pains. Hedge listened to chest sounds. He said, "A funny murmur." Goldson listened and said, "No, it's not what you think it is." He and Hedge discussed the sound. Finally

Goldson said, "OK, but I think when you get the cardiogram and a consult, you'll see that I'm right." [June 3, 1964]

I met Hedge on the ward, with the woman he had admitted a few days ago. I asked him who was right, he or Goldson. "Oh," he said, "Goldson was right. It wasn't what I thought. The AR can always teach you a thing or two. Now he'll be hard to handle. He'll think he was right this time, so he has to be right next time. He knows what he wants done, but as long as the guy is reasonable, you can discuss it with him." [June 7, 1964]

The intern who disagrees with a resident is asserting his equality, implying that he knows as much medicine as the resident does. A resident need not deny the intern's claim by telling him this is not so. His opinion is probably the more informed of the two, and he expects that this will be confirmed by the consulting physician. Since most differences of opinions are resolved in favor of residents, interns are reminded that they are still not equal, but inferior in knowledge. The residents can still teach them a thing or two they need to know. By tolerating differences of opinions and submitting to a third party, residents do nothing to subvert an egalitarian relationship with interns, but replenish their depleted power by demonstrating that they still have something to exchange.

The assistant resident supervises medical care. He oversees and coordinates such work as taking complete histories, doing thorough physical examinations, making diagnoses, and providing treatment. If an assistant resident can dictate a discharge summary indicating that everything that should have been done for the patients on his ward was done, he has done his job well. To discharge his responsibility, he needs the cooperation of interns who do the actual work. To gain and keep it, he tacitly agrees to provide interns with a variety of services.

I was on the ward talking with Prentice [intern] when Harris [intern] motioned me over to tell me that Seeling, the new assistant resident, had called a meeting with the interns. "He's taking over the ward today," explained Harris, "and he wants to tell us how he's going to run it. Each AR has a little different idea of how things should be. Though they are our patients, he has the say."

We met in the conference room on the third floor of the Peabody Building. "I just want to say a few things," Seeling told us. "If I wait until we all have the time to meet, it would never get done. I think making it a formal meeting gets it over with."

Harris asked him if anybody arranged to get slides for the laboratory. "I would think," replied Seeling, "we should have no trouble getting supplies. I could always arrange in the past to get what was needed." "So," said Harris, "arrange already." Seeling made a note. "Sorry I'm late," said Prentice as he entered the room, "but I had to attend to some things." "Bullshit!" said Harris. "You were eating." "More shit," said Prentice, as he lay back on a bed in the room. "Wake me when this meeting is over," he said. Seeling asked if the students were coming to the meeting. "They have work to do," Harris told him.

"I just want a few minutes," Seeling said, "to explain how I would like to run things. It will still be your ward, but I saw some things on the other service that I don't want repeated here. I think they can be avoided. First, I think it's best if we all do our own jobs. I will be running around to get things, and I want you to make sure things get done. That won't leave me much time to do my work. I have to write my notes so we know what we are doing when we go over the charts. If I don't do that when I should, I'll never get it done. I don't think we should have chart conferences every day. You know what you're doing. So, how about every other day?" Everyone agreed. "That'll give us more time to do our work," said Harris. "Also," said Seeling, "I'll try to work up every patient so I'm in touch with what you are doing. OK?" "If you want to," replied Prentice, "that'll be good. Harry [the previous AR] was good that way. He would just jump in there with us. That would be great. I thing it would be a big help." "OK," said Seeling. "I don't know if I'll be able to work up every patient, but I will work up most. I don't want to be doing all the pneumonias, but I will do the more-than-routine patients. I won't make long notes. I'll make short comments on the charts. They are still your patients, but I do want to know what's going on. I'll also start rounds on the dot. If we start evening rounds at 5, there should be no reason why we shouldn't finish in time for you to have dinner. Any questions?" No one had questions. [April 19, 1965]

Interns resent the assistant resident who is late for evening rounds, since he may cause them to miss their evening meal. They also resent a resident who does not work up patients. Often they have two or more admissions at the same time and cannot work up each one immediately. A willing assistant resident can make the admission process easier. Furthermore, interns think that the assistant resident cannot discuss patients unless he has worked them up himself. Interns on Seeling's ward, then, obviously appreciated his promises to them. He also promised that he would run around to make sure that things got done. The assistant resident can do many things to help interns.

I met Huptman [assistant resident] at the elevator. He was carrying a patient chart. When I asked him whose chart it was, he said, "I've just gotten this chart by real devious and complicated means. The patient was admitted, but no one knew he had previously been a patient. We had no records for him, though he insisted he had been here before. I went over to records and found out he had been at the outpatient department. His chart was being held up for insurance reasons. I ran down and got it away from them." He and I rode the elevator up to the ward. We entered the laboratory and Huptman handed the chart to Eliot [intern]. "Where," exclaimed Eliot, "did you get this? This is a real pearl," he told me. "I can really use this." "It's all in knowing how," said Huptman. [June 29, 1965]

I was running to the wards with Booth [assistant resident]. We were in the House Officer's Building when he got a telephone call from Kaufmann [intern], asking for help. It was late at night, and as we passed the mailboxes we saw Harris [intern who was the night float] stuffing consult requests in the boxes. "What's up?" he asked. "I thought I'd get this out of the way early." Booth told him that Kaufmann had more than he could handle. "Why don't you," he asked, "go over and give him a hand? The two of you can probably handle things on the ward. I'm going over to pick up a patient of his, the

MI that just came in. I'll take care of her for him, and you can help him with the other admissions." Later I was with Kaufmann. "Thank God," he said. "He'll keep an eye on her. Having a float is a big help, but a good resident is a godsend. He can always be of help. They don't have to do all they do, but residents always seem to be right guys. If you honestly try to do your job and they know you are, you can expect help." [January 7, 1965]

Residents need not do these favors but when they do, they place the interns in their debt. Interns appreciate what residents do for them.

"The assistant residents," Koren [intern] told me, "are usually available and always ready to be of help. They share their experience and are also willing to do things for you. A resident, for example, might run down with a requisition you didn't have time to deliver or pick up some pictures for you. They do things like that for you. So I have no complaints about residents. They have always been around and been a great help. Know what else? Not one of them has taken advantage by pushing his own ideas, his own way of doing things on me. They also share what they read with me. It's been a good relationship." [June 1, 1965]

As these comments suggest, assistant residents do the reading that interns have no time for.

Hertman [intern] entered the laboratory. Goldson asked how Mrs. Jones, Hertman's patient, was doing. "Not bad," said Hertman. "That article I mentioned to you," Goldson said, "is on the desk. You want to read it. It's only a couple of pages long, but I outlined the clinical part. It's only about a page and won't take too long to read." Hertman thanked him. "Hey," said Kaufmann, "I want to read it too." [May 3, 1965]

In addition to finding articles that are pertinent, assistant residents also share their knowledge of the literature on the wards. An intern told me:

The library here doesn't mean anything to me, because I don't get a chance to read that much. You have to have time to

read. Who has time? I have too much to do to take the time
to read everything written about a problem one of my patients
has. Now and then I'll look at an article or read a journal.
But most of the time I depend on other people. I depend a lot
on the assistant resident and other people like the visit to keep
me up on the medical literature. [December 23, 1964]

Interns believe that everybody who can keeps up with medical
literature, so they don't hesitate to ask residents to keep them
informed:

We were making rounds. The first patient was an epileptic.
After Prentice [intern] examined him, he turned to Mayer
[assistant resident] and asked, "What's in the literature? Anything I should know?" "I have an article on the treatment of
epilepsy," said Mayer, "but the authorities don't say anything
about this kind of seizure." "Good," said Prentice, "then I
don't have to read it." We moved on to the next patient, a
diabetic. Harris [intern] examined this patient. When he
finished, he asked, "How about the diabetic literature? You
must be up on the studies." "I have a couple at home," said
Mayer, "and there is one real good article, but I don't remember the exact title. The studies are inconclusive, because
it's difficult to maintain controls. You can't control on enzyme
differences, types of patients, and things like that." The
senior resident nodded. "I'll bring the article in, but it may
not be of much help to you." [July 17, 1964]

One final circumstance serves to maintain the relationship between intern and resident as social exchange. After the middle
of the year, interns are looking back on the internship and
forward to their residencies. Most of them will stay on at the
hospital and assume the positions now occupied by assistant
residents. Thus it behooves them to acknowledge that the ward
is the responsibility of the resident and that interns must cooperate with him. In the interest of future gain, they accept
the principles that support the position of assistant residents.
To do otherwise would subvert power that will soon be theirs.

THE SOCIAL ORGANIZATION OF THE HARVARD MEDICAL SERVICES

A hospital is usually thought of as a hierachy, with rules defining the rights, obligations, and duties of each position. The various positions are also assumed to carry differential status and power. If this were so, the intern, with the status of a physician, would have the power to implement the treatments he selects and to get the services he needs for patient care.

The rules at Boston City Hospital, however, are vague. They do not set forth the rights and obligations of those who must work together to care for patients. Furthermore the rules are not always binding. For example, the name of a patient should not be placed on the danger list unless his condition is truly serious. This is a rule. Because a telegram must be sent to the next of kin and a clergyman notified each time a patient is placed on the danger list, the hospital's administrators try to keep the list short to cut down on clerical work. But an intern can always get a porter to transport a patient whose name is on the danger list. Therefore, to expedite transportation, interns readily put patients on the danger list, which they couldn't do without the complicity of residents and nurses. The rules for obtaining other services can just as easily be circumvented with the tacit approval of nurses, clerks, and technicians. Hospital rules are less important than a shared understanding of how things should be done.

The organization that is the Harvard Medical Services consists of relationships negotiated and established on the basis of social exchange. What I have said about Boston City Hospital does not imply that the situation there is atypical. On the contrary, the ignorance of interns who begin training at any hospital makes social exchange characteristic of the internship. The hospitals and the medical services they operate cannot be explained by a conventional medical model, with the physician in complete authority. The hospital must be examined as a locale where personnel, mostly but not exclusively professionals, are enmeshed in a negotiative process by which they accomplish their ends and the stated purpose of the institution.[5]

The diplomacy, bargaining, and improvisation I observed could, of course, be attributed to unique conditions at Boston City. This hospital is operated under the auspices of the city. Most others are not. Three medical schools share its facilities. The hospital is old and dilapidated. The shortage of nurses and other paramedical personnel is more serious here than at other hospitals, particularly teaching institutions. All of these conditions may call for somewhat devious dealings. My contention, however, is that bargaining is typical of the relationships among hospital personnel anywhere, and that diplomacy and improvisation are simply part of social exchange.

Studies of other hospitals support this position. Sociologists who studied the Michael Reese Hospital in Chicago, for example, suggested that an approach emphasizing negotiation would be useful because it directs attention to exchanges among personnel as well as to hierarchical prescriptions of rights, obligations, and duties.[6] Such an approach to the hospital permitted explanation of what I observed to be the organization of the Harvard Medical Services at Boston City Hospital.

What must be further explained, however, is why social exchange was so characteristic of what I observed. The answer is that the Harvard Medical Unit's elite status not only affects the work that interns must do but also establishes the conditions under which they must work.

The work itself has little to do with the elite careers that many interns will eventually have in medicine. They must, however, do that work because the Unit has implicitly contracted with the hospital to provide patient care.

The freedom to do the research on which it bases its status as an elite segment of medicine, the fact that Harvard chooses to maintain the Unit at Boston City Hospital, requires that interns be concerned with social exchanges. A city hospital with numer-

5. See Anselm Strauss and others, "The Hospital and Its Negotiated Order," in Eliot Friedson, ed., *The Hospital in Modern Society* (New York, Free Press, 1963), p. 167.
6. Strauss and others, "The Hospital and Its Negotiated Order."

ous patients having a variety of medical problems is a local place to locate the Unit, but it also places interns in a setting with less than adequate facilities and insufficient ancillary personnel. Simply, the location of the Unit in Boston City Hospital best serves the elite purposes of Harvard physicians, but requires interns to spend a great deal of their time running around and necessitates the process of social exchange.

8. Perspectives on Work

INTERNS face the problem of participating in academic activities when the demands of providing patient care require almost all their time. They must therefore coordinate their academic activities with their work, and develop a perspective to guide their actions toward that end. This requires them to define their situation, set goals for themselves in it, and evolve a rationale that legitimizes their activities during the year.[1]

The situation, however, is not the same throughout the year. At first the interns' most salient problem is mastery of their work. Their initial perspective therefore expresses a set of opinions about their responsibility to do the work of an internship,

1. A detailed explanation of the concept of perspective and extensive use of it for analytical purposes is reported in Howard S. Becker, Blanche Geer, Everett C. Hughes, and Anselm L. Strauss, *Boys in White* (Chicago, University of Chicago Press, 1961). My use of the concept is as defined by Becker and his collaborators: A perspective is a plan of action tacitly approved by a group of people in a problematic situation or setting.

and is strongly influenced by the opinions of others at the hospital. After they have learned the ropes, they are somewhat less preoccupied with the mechanics of their work, having by then mastered much of it. When they are familiar enough with the situation to know what is actually required of them, they are more or less free to determine their own level and direction of effort. They then tacitly evolve an operating perspective, or standard of performance, made up of opinions about the relative value of the work required of them and the criteria they use to determine what they need and need not do.

THE INITIAL PERSPECTIVE

Interns have a great deal of work to do. The long hours on the wards and in the laboratory are recognized as part of the job. Even the physicians who select interns, concerned as they are with class standing, letters of recommendation, and the other evidence of academic success, acknowledge the almost exhausting amount of work interns have to do. A common description of a promising applicant: He looks like he'll be able to do the work.

All medical students spend some time at hospitals where they watch interns at work, so they shouldn't be surprised at the work load they themselves encounter. They are surprised, though, if not actually overwhelmed, to discover just how much there is to do.

> In the laboratory I asked Pearson how he felt at the end of his second day at the hospital. "Well, I thought most of what I would be doing would be preparing me to be a physician. I didn't think I would be doing so much lab work and as much nursing as I am. You have to spend a great deal of time doing those things. I knew I had to do some of them, but I didn't think it would take so much time. I guess I just didn't know how much I would have to do. I'm glad to be here. I'm doing what I wanted to be doing. It's just a little overwhelming. I'll get used to it." [June 29, 1965]

Most are also surprised at the kind of work they must do and see in it little relevance to their future careers.

When I asked Prema how he thought the things he was doing would prepare him to be a doctor, he said, "I guess it doesn't, really. It prepares you to take care of your patients, I guess. A lot of the things I do, I guess I'll not have to do if I go into practice. It does teach you how to be efficient, I guess. It will help by giving me confidence. It's really hard to say. I don't know. It's just a lot of hard work." Another intern, Zucker, said, "Things aren't too bad. We're all a little tired, but I think we'll get things straightened out. I wish I had time to think. Everything seems to be running into everything else. I'm not sure how, but things are going, and little by little, it's coming. I just want to get all my work done." [July 1, 1965]

Since they cannot say why, interns "guess" that this kind of work will contribute in some way to their becoming competent physicians. They are so busy those first few weeks that they have no time to think about it. They simply accept that the work must be done for some good reason. Interns do not hesitate to talk about the importance of working, but they are hard put to justify their particular assignments.

I was sitting at a table with Perkins [intern], eating lunch. Perkins shook his head and said, "It's not the physical work. I'm big. I feel right now physically able to do more work and get with it, but it's the emotional strain." Gallagher [assistant resident] joined us at the table. Perkins nodded to him, saying, "If I were him, I'd be mad at me all the time. I just make stupid mistakes, and foul everything up. I just don't seem to get things straight, and so I don't get things done. It's important to get all your work done and I'm not doing that, I'm not getting my work done." Gallagher said, "Stop worrying about it. You need your strength." Perkins shrugged and said, "I'm strong enough, but am I smart enough to do the work?" Gallagher: "That has nothing to do with you." Perkins: "I know, it's the place. It's this place. Each place has its own style of wardmanship, but I'm just not finding out what it is." Gallagher reassured him, "Don't worry about it." Perkins shrugged. He finished his meal and said, "I'd better get back to work."
As we left the dining room, he turned to me and said,

"I'm really tired. I try to do all the procedures for each patient. That doesn't work. I decided now that I'm going to organize. I'm going to pull all procedures that are the same together and do all of them at once. I don't see any other way of doing it all." I asked him why he had to do it at all. He said, "You have to get your work done. That's a good enough reason." [July 5, 1965]

Most interns are not so desperate as this one, but all will insist that it is important to do all the work.

Leishman [intern] said: "You go through an experience that means something. I guess I always expected to have responsibility. You don't really know what it is to have responsibility. It always looks so good and easy until you really find out what it means. I really didn't think that these things would take that much time. Everything we do takes time. I didn't think I'd have to spend so much time doing lab work, dressings, and all that. I just didn't realize that this is what responsibility is."

I asked Huber [another intern] if he agreed with Leishman. Huber answered, "I think that the thing you have to be is compulsive and get your work done. Spend every morning with the visit or at conference and the rest of the time working. I expected to spend most of my time taking care of patients, and that's what I wanted responsibility for." I asked him what he did have responsibility for and he replied, "We have the responsibility for seeing that everything gets done. That's our job." [July 5, 1965]

Interns don't just say they should get everything done; they actually try to do it. They stay at the hospital until all hours of the night, examining patients, carrying out medical procedures, doing laboratory tests, and writing it all down in the patients' charts. Early the next morning they are back, finishing last-minute chores before another day begins. As if this pace weren't grueling enough, they try to do all their academic work as well, though they may sleep through some of the lectures and conferences.

Apparently, then, interns' initial perspective includes not only a lot of work but an aim to do it all. What is not obvious is why they set themselves such a goal. If they saw clearly that what they were doing would make them better doctors, their relentless drive would not be hard to understand. But they do not see how their present work prepares them for the future. Why, then, even after they have some time to think about it, do they try to do it all?

There are, of course, many possible answers. They may do it at first because they think they have to in order to earn a good residency. This is partly the answer. The most naive of interns know that patients must be cared for and that interns are used to doing so. They also know the implied reward: By doing the work they obligate Harvard physicians to assist them with future problems and decisions. The implicit agreement between interns and the Harvard physicians is: Do the work now, and we will take care of you. Interns soon learn, however, that they are less visible than they supposed to people who could affect their careers. No matter what their ultimate career goal, the immediate problem is simply to get through the year. An intern could, if he wanted to, do less work without seriously jeopardizing his opportunity for a good residency. The making of a good record, therefore, does not entirely explain why interns set themselves a goal of doing all their work.

At the beginning of the year, interns are influenced not so much by implicit rewards as by their definition of the working situation. They try to keep up with all the work because it is their responsibility. They apply the idea of medical responsibility to the situation they are in and conclude that as responsible interns they must do it all.

Having been told that responsibility for patients is the hallmark of a physician, medical students look forward to their internships because they will have such responsibility. Much of what interns have to do, however, could be done by someone else, not necessarily a physician. To justify doing this sort of work, interns incorporate the idea of responsibility into their initial perspective. As students, interns admit, they thought of medical responsibility as the management of patient's illnesses. They soon learn that the welfare of their patients requires more than the diagnosis and treatment of disease. Responsibility, they discover, encompasses not only medical problems but also management of the total hospital situation to gain the maximum benefit for the patients. Thus they find themselves doing nursing, laboratory, and administrative, as well as purely medical, tasks.

> I think the shortcomings of this hospital—you know, not enough nurses, all the things you have to do for yourself, and all that—are made up for by all the good things about the hospital. . . . you do get responsibility. It's a lot of hard work, but you do feel like you're doing something, accomplishing something. You're doing something, differently now as an intern than as a student. As a student, you don't realize that responsibility isn't only for medical care, but it's for all the other things too. You're responsible for all the scut as well as taking care of patients. Even when you know what you have to do and how to do it, it's still a lot of hard work. It's just time consuming to do everything you have to do, but that's responsibility. [July 8, 1965]

Assistant residents play a key role in fostering the interns' whole-hog attitude toward responsibility:

> Huber [intern] and Goode [assistant resident] started rounds and went right on seeing patients through visiting hours. As we went from patient to patient, Huber listed everything that had to be done for each one. Goode wanted to talk. It wasn't too long ago that he and I stood on this ward laughing at the travel posters the interns' wives had put on the wall to add some color. As we were reminiscing, Huber kept motioning us on, saying, "Let's get through rounds." Goode retorted, "Don't tell me let's go. Go on yourself and examine the patient. She's your responsibility." He turned to me and laughed and we followed Huber. At the bedside of each patient, Goode told Huber what had to be done, and Huber added to his list. At the last patient, Goode said, "I'm going to be a real illegitimate child about these patients. We have to record the medications. Either you record nothing at all, which is unthinkable to me, or you record everything. We have to agree on this." Goode looked at Huber's list and cautioned him to get everything down. Then they finished rounds. [July 5, 1965]

In so defining interns' responsibility, the assistant resident prescribes a level and direction for their efforts. Goode in effect told Huber what he must do and how much of it he must expect to get done; he was not to stop short of trying to do it all.

The interns' initial perspective developed in their first weeks at the hospital may be summed up this way:

1. An internship entails an almost overwhelming amount of work.

2. The work is hard, it is important, because it is somehow relevant to becoming a good physician, and, for numerous reasons, will stand the intern in good stead in medicine.

3. Although all the work is not obviously valuable experience, it is the intern's responsibility to do it. He is not privileged to limit himself to caring for patients.

4. If an intern is not getting his work done, he must find a way to do it. He must organize his effort so as to do everything he has to.

THE REALITY OF WORK

Most interns give up all their leisure time. Though they are permitted, for example, to use the Harvard athletic facilities, few do so. As one said:

> I never used my Harvard athletic card. I may have played indoor tennis a couple of times, but never got a chance to do any of the other stuff. It was disappointing. I really do enjoy athletics. I really missed having the time to do some of the things I was looking forward to, but when I first came here, I just jumped right in doing everything. Now, I want to get out of here so I can go home earlier, about 8:00 or so. I never had any time before, because I would stay here until 11:00 or later trying to do my work. [May 19, 1965]

Interns who are engaged have little time to spend on dates.

> Benson [assistant resident] told us that he and his wife took short trips to the South Shore, but never had time to go all the way to Cape Cod. Smith [intern] joined us at the table, asking Butler [intern], "Is your honey coming in this

week?" Butler: "Yes, I told her to come in, and I think we'll get out even if I don't have my work finished." Smith laughed. "That's all right. You should finish your Thursday and Friday patients by midnight on Saturday. That'll give you Sunday to tangle. That's not too bad. One day." Butler, also laughing, said, "You're not kidding. It will work out that way." [July 27, 1964]

Married interns have little time to spend with their wives.

I asked Smith [intern] how his wife was. He told me that she was staying with her parents. "It had to be done. She thought it would be best. I'm on the wards most of the time and have little time to be home. She deserted me." "How do you feel about that?" He said, "Well, I'm compulsive about my work. She doesn't mind that. I guess I can't mind her being practical. It was a good idea, since I have so much to do here at the hospital." [July 31, 1964]

Though an intern may feel guilty about neglecting his wife, he nevertheless stays at the hospital.

Smith said, "She's back now. Got back yesterday. I'm on tonight and have to stay here. I felt a little guilty last night. It was her first night back. She gives me no gas about it, but I did want to be home. I had this patient that was just on the line, really sick. I couldn't see any way clear and had to stay around until about 11:00. It's a good thing she was gone the first week, and I wasn't torn between her and work." [August 4, 1964]

During the first month or so interns try to do everything they can. When they do not have the time, they make it by giving up their leisure or sacrificing family life, though they are not happy about these choices.

Concerned that some tests scheduled by someone at the Harvard School of Public Health would be confused with my study, I went looking for Donnelly, the intern who reacts most vehemently to such demands on interns' time. I asked him if he had a few minutes to talk. He nodded, "I rushed through lunch, so I'm in no real hurry." I asked if he had seen the memorandum about the test. He had not. I gave him my copy. He read it and looked up, saying, "Well, I had a good night of sleep, so I guess it won't upset me too much. Don't worry about it. I don't think any of the guys think it's your fault. I've never seen a place like this. They really push the interns around. They don't really know what we have to do. The intern is the only one who does the work around here. You can't trust the student to do any work, and you can't trust the nurse. It's easier to weigh patients yourself, draw blood, take the patient over to X-ray, just do everything yourself. You ask the nurse to do it, you've got to check and make sure it gets done. I know what'll happen after this test. We'll all be here late at night. Things like that are a pain. You know, like today. A friend called and said how about a swim. I said sure. I rushed through lunch and wanted to get to clinic early so I would have time for a swim. Then this comes up. Well, I have the time, so it isn't too bad. If I didn't have the time, I still would want to do it. I think we all try to do everything they want us to do. I just go along and try to get all my work done." [August 19, 1964]

Like Donnelly, all interns try at first to do everything that is defined for them as part of their job. And it seems that everything is. Even participation in studies like mine was presented as a *"responsibility* to encourage the advancement of knowledge." Interns are told that they should be willing to do all these things because it is their responsibility. After a time, however, they begin to realize that achieving such a goal is impossible and to question the wisdom of some of the things they have to do.

On my way to the Peabody Building I met Katz, the intern who had been admitting patients yesterday. He raised a hand, shook his head, and said, "I was up all night. I had one [a patient] who kept me on the go all night. I can't sleep very well over there [motioning to the Peabody Building]. I'll sleep better there [pointing to the House Officer's Building.]" I asked him what was going on. "A conference, a student conference. I'm going to pass it up. You know, you can't do everything and go to everything, I'll get sick." I told him he didn't have to explain to me. Katz shrugged, "I know, I know. But you feel so guilty if you cut out on something. I don't get much out of them, but you just feel you have to go. Maybe, they're important, but I need my sleep more." [August 9, 1964]

Katz did not, in fact, get to sleep.

I was at the conference, sitting near the door so I could see what was going on down the hall as well as in the room. Marlo and Howell [interns] were both dozing, eyes closed and chin on chest. Katz did not attend the conference but he did not get to bed. I could see him going in and out of the doors to the laboratory. He had urine samples, test tubes, and was carrying patient charts, obviously working.

Interns who try to make time to do everything they feel they should have little time for sleep. Staying late at the hospital gets the work done, but lack of sleep makes it difficult to get through the next day. The need for sleep marks the beginning of a change in perspective. They do not abruptly abandon their initial perspective, but gradually take up a new one as they lose more and more sleep. They begin to realize that, try as they will, they are not getting all their work done. Then they get discouraged. No matter how hard or long they work, they do not manage to attend to all their patients, do all the necessary laboratory work, participate in visiting rounds, and attend the scheduled conferences.

THE OPERATING PERSPECTIVE [2]

After a time, then, the interns alter their perspective as they redefine their situation.

2. My distinction between the initial perspective and the operating perspective is based on the rationale presented in Becker and others, *Boys in White,* and interns did evolve plans of action similar to those of students in medical school. There was, for example, an initial effort by interns to "do it all," which was much the same as the effort of students to "learn it all." Also, like medical students, interns realize that it all cannot be done and that such a perspective is impractical, requiring them to evolve another plan of action. The evolution of perspectives described by Becker and others was also characteristic of interns, so the presentation of data pertaining to interns' level and direction of effort is organized in much the same way as the data presented in *Boys in White.*

During work rounds, I noticed that interns were not staying with the group, as they had done at the beginning of the year. Yesterday Hartman left to do some laboratory work. Today Benson left in the middle of work rounds to prepare his presentation for visiting rounds. This is something they've started within the last month. [September 9, 1964]

Hartman later explained the change and gave some insight into the new perspective that was evolving.

When I asked if things had changed, Hertman said, "I think so, but I couldn't say how. Maybe it's just knowing you have to work 18 hours a day. That's the way you come to see it. Just 18 hours a day of problems of patient care." I asked why he was spending less time on work rounds. He said, "Do you think so? I think I spend as much time on rounds. Sometimes I have something I have to do so I'm late or leave early, but that's only if my work won't wait. I don't spend as much time at conferences, I think. If anything has changed, that has. I guess they're not as important as I thought they would be. I don't see them as having much to do with what I'm doing. A month ago, I wouldn't miss them, but now I do whenever my patients get to be too much."

I asked how his patients got to be too much. He answered, "You know, here even six or seven patients are too much. I've got enough to do with them and my patients at clinics. The conferences are OK, but if they're not on something I'm interested in, I'll forget it all. Just take care of your patients first, that's the ticket." [September 9, 1964]

Participation in academic activities is the first phase of interns' activity to change as they begin to moderate their efforts.

I entered the laboratory and was grabbed by Taggert [intern]. I kicked back and hit his shins. Laughing, he asked Cutler for help. Cutler just stood there laughing. He looked very thin, as if he had lost 20 pounds. He was chubby before. We all laughed and started for the conference room. Taggert took off his coat, but did not come into the room with us. He went to work in the laboratory instead. When I asked him why he had missed the conference, he said, "I've got too much to do. You can't do it all. Something has to give, and

I can't get behind on my work. You don't miss much when you miss one of those conferences and I can use the time better to do what I have to do on the wards." [September 10, 1964]

As interns become more and more involved with patient care, they conclude that this work deserves priority over their own activities. Occasionally this choice conflicts with the wishes of those in authority.

> We were making rounds on the ward when a nurse called for help with a patient who had been admitted for a myocardial infarct. The man had never been in a hospital before and was afraid of physicians. We all rushed into his room. May and Kingston [interns] were working over the patient, attempting resuscitation. The drama of the situation was increased because the oxygen equipment was leaking and could not be repaired while the interns were trying to save the patient. Everyone was doing something—preparing medications, resuscitating, trying to fix the equipment. A senior resident said, "You're going to have to strip your team down somehow. Decide who should stay, and the others can go. You have May and a student. A nurse too. That's about all you'll need. No?" The senior resident had previously asked if the assistant resident was going to go to coffee rounds with the associate director of the Harvard Services. The assistant resident said he preferred to stay. Now he asked the interns if they were going to the morning conference. They said they wanted·to stay. He said: "There's a cardiac conference going on now and you're a half-hour late."
>   The interns left the room reluctantly, but did not go directly to the conference. They stopped at patients' beds, in the laboratory, or at the nurses station. When a laboratory technician stopped the intern I was with and asked, "Are you very busy now?" he shook his head. "Do you need some blood?" he asked. She said, "I do, on Mr. Jones, but if you're busy I can come back later." He said, "I'm not too busy, but I was on my way to a conference. I drew some blood this morning. Will that do?" The technician said it would not, so he went to draw some more blood. As he was going, he turned to me and said, "I'd rather go for coffee, but I guess I'll go over to the conference. I'll only be a minute, so wait for me and I'll walk over with you." [August 29, 1964]

When the senior resident told the assistant to strip the team, I thought he was trying to get some of us out of the room. This, however, was not the case. He wanted everyone who possibly could to go to the conference. A similar incident occurred the next day.

> The patient who required emergency care yesterday was being presented to the visiting physician. Kingston explained what had happened during the emergency, then admitted he did not know why it had happened. The interns were discussing this with the visiting physician when the senior resident walked into the room, saying, "I hate to interrupt, but the chief resident says there's a conference on cancer of the breast to which you are all invited. It's going on now. We are all urged to attend." The interns continued to discuss the patient. After a few minutes, the senior resident said, "Why don't those who are caring for this patient stay and discuss him with the visiting physician, but the rest of us go over to the conference?" He turned to walk away, but stopped and said to the visiting physician, "I want him [pointing to Kingston] to get as much out of you as possible. Naturally, your opinions are important and we want them." Then he left the room.
>
> I went after him and asked: "Why urge the interns to attend this conference?" He said: "I think those who are taking care of the patient should stay, because no matter how many books they read or how many conferences they attend, what they will remember is the patients they are caring for. I think that this is the heart of teaching, but the conference is with a new man who is joining the staff, and this is a good way to introduce him. This is the best time to have the conference, noon on Friday. It's just that the conference cuts into what they want to do. They knew about it. They had a notice about a week ago." Most of the interns followed us over to the conference. [August 21, 1964]

Incidents like these made me aware of the gradual change in the interns' perspective. Whereas they had at first made every effort to attend scheduled conferences, often knowing they would only have to return later to finish their work, they now chose to remain with their patients whenever there was a timing conflict. Other, more subtle, changes also emerged.

One of these was in their reading habits. All interns who were questioned before coming to the hospital said they expected to do a great deal of reading. Many stressed the importance of keeping up with the professional literature. Once on the job, however, interns found little time for reading.

> We were in the lab, sitting and talking, I asked Harper [intern], "How busy have you been?" Harper: "I've only had one admission since I've been here. I've been lucky. I haven't been as busy as the others. I still don't know what's what. Just learning where things are and how to get them takes a while." Harper had said before coming to the hospital that he thought he would have time to read and that it was absolutely necessary for him to do so. I asked about his reading, and he said, "I may have time later on. It's like everything else, you make time for it. The work I have to do is something I only thought I knew about. I knew I had to work hard, but I didn't know what hard was. I just had no idea. I kept thinking to myself, I know there's a routine here somewhere, and once I learn it, everything will be OK." [July 1, 1965]

Interns read when they can. Although they try to read everything pertinent to their patients' problems, they do not think it possible to read just to keep up with the medical literature. They find this out quickly, after a week or so.

> English told me he was depressed because he didn't have time to do everything he had to. I retorted laughingly saying, "That's responsibility." He then added, "But not this much. There you are, and you have to know how and what to do." When I asked what he had been doing, he said, "I spend most of my time running around . . . You don't really know what it is to have responsibility. I didn't think these things would take so much time. Everything we do takes a lot of time. It takes all day to get your work done. I don't even have time to read. [He had expected to read a lot during the year]. I didn't expect to have to do all this running around.

I didn't think I'd have to spend so much time doing lab work, dressing, and all that. I just didn't expect this. I didn't realize that this is what our responsibility would be for. When you think of patient care, it's not in terms of these things. Yes, I thought I'd have time to keep up with the literature. Forget it. It's not possible when you have all these other things to do. Now I have to depend on others." [July 5, 1965]

When the interns found it impossible to maintain a high level of academic effort and still do all they had to for their patients, they called into question the very idea of responsibility. "We are responsible for our patients," they began to say, "and maybe that's all we should be responsible for."

Interns might simply redefine responsibility to exclude everything not directly related to patient care, thus implying they consider academic activities less important. This would logically lead, however, to defining the internship as nothing more than a lot of hard work to be endured in order to earn certification. While this may actually be so, interns cannot accept such a definition of their situation. To do so would acknowledge that learning is less important than work and deny the educational benefit of serving the internship. Interns think of medicine as a body of knowledge they must learn. Their efforts, they believe, must be directed as much toward learning as toward doing their work. Thus, a perspective that does not view the internship as a learning situation is of no use to them.

Faced with the problem of reconciling the conflicting demands of learning and of work, interns reduce their participation in formal learning activities. But these are exactly the activities that justify the internship as a learning experience. Since the value they place on the internship lies in the interrelation of learning and work, interns must evolve a perspective that permits them to redirect their efforts without subverting that relationship. Hence they must establish the educational value of the work they have decided has to come first. They accomplished this by introducing aspects of learning into their work. The work itself assumes meaning in terms of its learning potential.

At first you say, "Boy, I'm not going to be able to handle all this." My own ignorance was frustrating at the beginning. All the frustrations that are a part of any internship also get you down. You know, you can't get an X-ray when you need it, or you can't find a chart, or they are all out of this or that when you need it, or they haven't got a drug you need, or the nurses aren't around. All this is frustrating. And you thought what you were going to be doing would all be important, so you tried to do it all. I think it kind of dawns on you gradually that all of it *isn't* important, just because you have responsibility for it. It's the learning of the realities of medicine. What's good is that you are sort of on your own, but the internship is so full and busy that there are really few dramatic times. Soon you realize that a lot of what you're doing doesn't have to be done. Not everything you do gives you experience. When you do your work you just get exposed to all kinds of problems. You get a tremendous amount of experience that way. I can't really point to any specific experiences, but an internship is just a whole lot of little experiences with patients by which you gain confidence. If you can do all your work here you just have to believe that you can take care of patients anywhere. [April 19, 1965]

To rationalize the shift in focus from formal study to patient care, interns invoke another idea common in medical education, the idea of clinical experience. "There are two ways of learning," they say, "from books and by seeing things for yourself." Work with patients offers the second type of learning. Thus interns legitimize their choice of a level ("you can't do it all") and a direction ("just take care of your patients first; that's the ticket") by stressing the value of clinical experience.

Dearborn had told me when he first came on the wards that the internship was just now a lot of hard work, "A lot of crap that somebody has to do." He said, "I'm enjoying myself. I don't try to do everythinug, like I did at first. I used to do everything I was told to do, but now I know what I have to do and what I can do without, because I don't get anything out of it." "What," I asked, "do you want out of what you're doing?" "I want as much experience as I can get. Next year [as an assistant resident] I'll have time to read and get some depth, but now I'm getting a lot of experience." Trying to be funny, I said, "Working less, but enjoying it more." He shook his head and said, "Hell no. I'm working my ass off, but I'm learning a lot of medicine." [November 20, 1964]

When interns incorporate the idea of clinical experience, they begin to assess the value of various activities by the experience they provide.

At visiting rounds the medical student presented a patient described as hypersensitive, dehydrated, and in acidosis. The student summarized the admission data and gave the course of his hospital stay. I asked Land what he thought about the patients. "Well, the results of the [lab] tests are contradictory. It's hard to know what to make of them. I don't know what to think. There was a great deal of discussion about the patient among the visiting physician, interns, and medical students. Ricks, an intern who had just come on the ward from a tour of the outpatient department, asked: "Is this a hyperthermal case?" Tucker, the intern responsible for the patient, said, "Doctor Ricks knows of a reference in the literature about hyperthermal cases." "I've had some time to read. In the December *Lancet* there was a study." He reported what he had read.

Another intern said: "I saw three of these cases when I was a student here, and they all died." Land said, "These cases aren't rare. There's another one around. I saw one last month too." "Let's take a look at the patient," said the visiting physician. We went along while Tucker examined his patient. The visiting physician suggested he continue treating the patient as he had been.

Land said, "I think the rounds were good today. There was a lot to get excited about. It was an important case." "What, I asked, "makes this an imortant case?" He told me it was important because it was not typical. "He's sick, and we have other people who have some of the problems he has, but you rarely see anyone with so many problems. You have to control all of his systems. You're keeping him alive . . ." Ricks, who was next to us, said, "You have to use your head on this one. There are so many things that could be wrong. You've got to think of all of them. It's like doing detective work, a great experience." Land said to me, "That's right. Today was good, because the case gives you exerience in diagnosis. You have a lot to do, but you think it over, talk about it, and learn a lot." [August 24, 1964]

Later that morning I asked the assistant resident why he had selected that particular patient to present to the visiting physician. He answered:

It's really a typical case, but more important, it offered an opportunity for learning, a chance for the intern to do a lot of different things. This patient makes a variety of demands on your skills and gives you a lot of experience you wouldn't otherwise get. [August 24, 1964]

At lunch, I talked to the senior resident about the case:

"What," I asked, "made today's case so important?" "There are a number of reasons," he said. "why it's an important case and why the interns get excited about it. This is a very sick patient, but we can do something for him. He also presents a wider range of problems, more of a challenge. It's just not routine patient care. He [the intern in charge] will remember this case, and the others will remember what they talked about. It's the involvement that's important. If they have to read, they will read, but otherwise you won't make the time to read. You're too busy taking care of your patients. This case offered Tucker a good opportunity to practice, to get experience. But Ricks, the intern who talked about the article on hypothermal damage, has a bookish approach to medicine. He had theory emphasized when he was a student, and he is carrying on the same way, or using the same approach here. Others are not like that. The others are more, I guess, learning by doing or applying what they learned." Brown [intern], who had joined us at the table, said, "I think it was a very good visit. I learned today more about electrolytes than I thought I would ever know." The senior resident turned to me and said, "You see, if he read it, he might not remember it, but when he learns it in terms of a patient, he will remember it." [August 24, 1964]

Interns, residents, and students all agree that the "more valuable" activities are those that offer broad experience. Visiting rounds are "good" when they center on patients with a variety of problems, and an "important case" is one that demands the doing of a variety of things. Activities of this sort, interns say, are "more valuable" than "book learning" or attending scheduled academic activity.[3] An intern told me:

> I've missed lots of conferences. I think I don't get too much out of the conference and get a lot more out of sitting by my patients and watching them, taking a pulse, or reading about a patient's disease. I'll learn a lot more that way. The thing is, who am I working for? I'm working for myself, that's who. [December 23, 1964]

Interns also use the idea of experience to excuse not reading the medical literature unless it pertains to the diseases of their patients. An intern said:

> It's important to read. Read every time you have an opportunity to, but if I took time to do a lot of reading, I probably would not have had the experience I have had. It would not have been enough to just read. To be a good doctor, I had to get the experience I did get. If I did take time to read, I wouldn't be doing my work. I read when it has something to do with my patients. [June 11, 1965]

The demands of routine work, however, make it impossible for interns to limit their efforts only to the "more valuable" activities. Even when an intern has an interesting case, his day-to-day work must still be his primary concern.

> I met Benson on the ward, changing a dressing. When I asked him what he thought of visiting rounds that day, he said, "I'm interested in metabolic problems, so this was a good day for me. We had to worry about the patient's metabolic state all the time. There are a whole range of things you could do for this guy, and you have to pick out the ones to do. I think that this is what makes this case interesting. I also don't have to

---

3. In *Boys in White* it was reported that students learn that practical experience is more valuable than book learning. Though students apparently come to such a conclusion during their clinical years, the belief in this tenet of medical education must persist during the internship or they would doubt the value of the work of an internship. Interns are therefore only acknowledging what they first came to believe as medical students, and using this tenet as a rationale for their adopted plan of action.

do the running around on this case. I could just sit back and listen and talk about the case. When you have to run around, you're caught up in the routine. You don't have the time to appreciate what's going on. You're so worried about treating the guy, you don't realize you are learning until later. This way, I can keep looking in on the guy, but Tucker has the responsibility." [August 24, 1964]

Interns want medical responsibility for an important case. They value highly the experience such responsibility gives them. But they no longer want the kind of total responsibility they initially accepted. "Who needs it?" an intern said to me. "Running around doing all those things doesn't add anything to what you already know, but taking care of a sick patient is a valuable experience." They will tell you, as I was told, that you have to get your work done, but the real learning comes in diagnosing and treating your patients. Though they are still concerned with the work they have to do, they no longer think all of it is valuable. The potential for clinical experience is the criterion on which they base their judgments. Discussing an "important case," for example, they consider educationally valuable because it does result in clinical experience even for those who have no responsibility for the routine work. When interns talk about these matters, it is obvious that they distinguish between responsibility as they first defined it and the more traditional idea of medical responsibility.

Interns continue to work at a high level, though they no longer consider everything they do important for learning. That is, they still do all the things that have to be done for their patients. Several things supply the impetus for this continued level of effort. First, the men do not want to obviously perform poorly. They want to do at least as well as the other interns; so they try to do as much of their own work as possible. Second, they accept the idea that medical responsibility includes an obligation to do for their patients anything that would not otherwise be done. The simple fact that there are not enough nurses on the wards requires the interns to work harder. Finally, their daily contact with residents encourages them to do as much of their work as they possibly can. Although they no longer want the sort of responsibility they initially envisioned, they do want medical responsibility as it is traditionally defined. They do not want to relinquish to residents the responsibility for patient care. Interns realize that residents can usurp their authority and that they control the means to assure that necessary work will be done. Thus the resident has a great deal to do with the interns' maintaining a high level of effort.

If interns admitted, however, that they were socially coerced to work at a high pitch, they would be denying the purpose of an internship; that is, they would be conceding that their efforts were not to further their own educational goals, but only to do the work that Harvard physicians wanted to be free of doing. Again, they need a rationale to justify working hard at things that do not, in their own opinion, furnish meaningful educational experiences.

Much as they used the idea of clinical experience to justify directing their effort toward patient care, they use the same idea to justify trying to do everything their patients need.

> We were in the laboratory. "This is the best slide I've ever seen," said Paretti [intern]. Moore [assistant resident] walked over and looked at the slide, asking, "What do you make of this?" "I don't know," said Paretti. "I think it's going to be difficult to diagnose." Moore said he didn't think it was pneumococcal pneumonia. "Yeah," said Paretti, "Well, you don't mind if I go ahead and treat him for pneumonia, do you?" Moore laughed and asked, "You don't believe me? I told you he doesn't have pneumonia." Paretti moaned, turned to me and said, "Such is the life of an intern. You can't even trust your assistant resident. If that's not pneumococcal pneumonia, I'll eat this slide. When I was at medical school I bet I didn't see two cases of pneumococcal pneumonia. Here, I can't remember how many I have seen. "Yes," said Moore, "and you know what? No matter how many you see, you learn from each one. Each one of them has something interesting about him. They're all a little bit different. You [turning to me] know it's true."
>
> "It's not only that," said Paretti, "the patient may be a little different or the course of the disease may not be the same, but everybody also brings something a little different

to the case. Even if you wanted to look at each case the same way, you have to listen to other people who are looking at it differently. That's what makes each patient an interesting case, and you learn something from every one of them. As long as you realize every case is different, you learn from each case. Each case is an experience in itself."

Moore, laughing said, "An old friend of mine used to say, 'Beware of the man who has seen a case,' and then he would say, 'I've seen a case of . . .' When someone is talking to you about a patient of yours, and he says 'I've seen a case of that': beware. I guess what I mean is that when you've seen a case you tend to treat what you think about it, rather than treat it as a paricular set of circumstances that you have to manage." Paretti said, "If you've seen a case, you might take it for granted, and not do everything you should for that particular patient." [April 7, 1965]

Interns often said that each case has some potential clinical experience, since each case has its unique course and consequences. Talk like Moore's and Paretti's also permits the resident to tell the intern that he must do everything for each and every patient, no matter how many times he has seen a case like the one he had admitted on the ward. "A good intern," an assistant resident told me, "is willing to approach a patient enthusiastically no matter how many times he has seen, for example, a stroke; when he gets another stroke, he doesn't just sulk, but goes ahead and does his work." On the matter of patient care, the interns' operating perspective does not conflict with the expectations of assistant residents.

> I think after a while it becomes difficult to say what you learn, but you do learn from each patient, if you pay attention to the patient. I think that each time you see one more case of something, you learn a little more, nothing specific but something that will make you more confident. You probably know a lot after the first time you see it, but new problems always come up, and you learn. That's why you have to approach each patient as a new experience. You know what you have to do, so you do it, but you are always looking for the idiosyncrasy you didn't see before. You may not have paid much attention to the little things the first few times you saw

a certain kind of case because you were worrying about the big things. Even if it looks just like another case, you can get more experience by doing your best for that patient. Well, maybe it is discouraging to have a lot of the same kinds of problems, but there is still a lot to be learned from them all. [June 2, 1965]

Many incidents and conversations recorded in my notes illustrate the importance interns place on patient care. These observations yield a picture of an operating perspective organized around the idea of clinical experience:

1. An intern cannot do everything that logically falls within his responsibility.

2. Since the work directly related to the problems of patients provides desirable clinical experience, an intern should direct his effort toward providing patient care.

3. An intern has medical responsibility for his patients, but must also accept some responsibility for other kinds of work related to their welfare.

4. An intern can make the time he needs to perform adequately at the second and third objectives above by reducing the effort he expends on academic activity.

THE CONGRUENCE OF PERSPECTIVES AND ELITE PURPOSE

Although in discussing perspectives I have treated responsibility and experience as distinct, discrete ideas, they are not mutually exclusive. Emphasizing the idea of responsibility does not preclude consideration of the idea of clinical experience in the initial perspective. Obviously, the reverse is also true. The idea of responsibility is an integral part of the operating perspective, despite its focus on clinical experience. Interns attempting to determine the relative value of the activities have recourse to these two ideas and use them to organize a way of thinking and acting at the hospital.

Given responsibility for the first time, they made maximum use of that idea in deciding what and how much they should do. The result was a perspective that set a goal of doing everything. This initial perspective led them to believe that everything they did was somehow important, and the idea of responsibility colored their judgment of every element of their immediate situation.

The reality of their work soon called into question the intern's definition of responsibility. There was, they came to think, such a thing as too much responsibility. There is no doubt that "too much responsibility" is but another way of saying "too much work." If there had been more interns to share the work, interns might have continued to define their responsibility in the same way throughout the year. As this point, no matter the reason, interns found other criteria for judging the value of their activities. Without denying responsibility, they concluded that a perspective organized primarily around it did not allow them to set a realistic level of effort and did not tell them where to direct their energies.

Interns must operate in the hospital, an institution organized for the purpose of providing service to patients. Thus they come to see patient care as their primary responsibility. The internship is supposedly a time of learning, particularly at a university-affiliated hospital. But to attend to their patients adequately, interns must divert some of their effort from academic pursuits. A perspective emphasizing the idea of clinical experience enables them to coordinate work with learning and legitimize their efforts chiefly to care for patients. It solves the problem of deciding what their level of effort should be ("get all the experience you can") and where that effort should be directed ("just take care of your patients").

The implications of the ideas around which perspectives are organized are important because of their effects on the direction of interns' efforts. If the initial perspective persisted, interns would divide their efforts between patient care and academic activity. The operating perspective is eminently more practical. Furthermore, it reduces the potential conflict between what interns want to do, what hospitals are in business to do, and what must be done if the Unit is to be a viable part of the hospital. The operating perspective I have described is a way of thinking and acting that does not conflict with the purpose of a hospital, and lends itself to the purpose of the Unit by permitting its physicians to devote themselves to research.

Interns come to define their situation and set themselves goals that make them valuable members of the medical labor force, without which the hospital could not stay in business. No matter how much interns complain, they do come to value exactly those activities they have to do. If they did not, they would not allow themselves to be used as they are in the hospital's division of labor, and more time and effort would be required of the Harvard physicians (a situation which would take those physicians away from activities more in keeping with their elite status).

Interns' eventual choice of perspective is not accidental. The people they must work with present and interpret the ideas of responsibility and experience. The prevailing practices and existing social norms preclude any other choice. By providing information from the medical literature, for example, the residents discourage interns' expending too much effort in reading by themselves. Assistant residents permit them to miss many conferences and lectures, thus indicating that patients are more important than academic activity. Paradoxical as it may seem, senior residents tolerate such action while taking steps to assure that interns will attend some conferences and lectures, "because no matter how many books they read, or how many conferences they attend, what they will remember is the patients they are caring for." The unofficial norms for intern's work support the prevailing practice of directing effort toward patient care. The fact that missing a conference is tolerated explains why interns choose to do so; that is, no social norm prohibits it.

There are, however, norms prohibiting reduction in effort expended on patient care. Failure to conform to these norms has consequences. If an intern does not do what he has to do for patients, it becomes obvious during work rounds. Since all interns know they are expected to have their work done, they do it. Many consider the failure to do everything necessary for a patient the most serious charge that could be made against an intern.

Only one of the interns I observed frequently violated this norm, and his behavior had a number of social consequences. First, he was the most unpopular intern. He had only a few friends, and these were interns on the other services, interns who did not have to work with him. His associates maintained their social distance, just short of ostracism. Second, he was not offered much help, a way of applying sanctions to enforce the norm for work.

> The assistant resident was on his way to the ward to see Clark. He asked Benson [intern], "How come you're not helping Clark? I thought that was your patient. How come you gave Clark such a good patient?" Benson said, "Well, he just wanted him so I gave him to him. I hope they take to each other. There's a lot to do." The assistant resident said, "They've taken to each other. Clark is down there on the ward now working his ass off." Benson nodded, turned to me and asked, "Do you want to walk over to X-ray with me?" When we returned we went to the ward where we met some visitors. Benson told me that Clark would talk with them. I asked if they were relatives of the patient Clark was working on. He said, "Yes, he's pretty sick. I don't know what Clark can do for him but Clark is going to spend a lot of time trying. I'm not a scut man, but I do expect interns to do most things that should be done, as they should on each and every job." [The implication was that Clark did not always do things as they should be done; therefore, Benson did not offer Clark any help, though we were on the ward. [April 7, 1965]

Since interns were encouraged to help one another, I didn't at first understand the assistant resident's tolerating Benson's implicit refusal to help Clark. When such behavior is a sanction for the enforcement of the norm, however, assistant residents apparently allow it. I observed only a few such incidents. Most interns do their work, though they did not want to be considered scut men who did or were expected to do things as they should be done. The existence of such a norm and the possibility of sanctions most certainly was an impetus for interns to expend their efforts on patient care.

In caring for patients, interns set a high level of effort. Their overall level, however, was less than what one would expect those in authority wanted. That is, they reduced considerably their participation in academic activity. Studies of other workers have described the phenomenon in which workers set production quotas lower than those expected by management. Sociologists would all agree that such quotas are the result of interaction among the workers. At Boston City Hospital the level of overall effort (quota) was, in fact, determined by interns, but management (assistant residents and residents) not only tolerated but possibly encouraged a lower level. While maintaining high expectations for patient care, they tacitly accepted, and even condoned neglect for academic activity. In this case, management apparently did not want maximum effort. The level of effort was less important than its direction.

The internship as I have described it is apparently a situation in which all that is supposed to be done cannot be done by interns. They must of necessity direct their effort toward doing what is most important and neglect what is less important— that is, evolve a perspective that requires a somewhat reduced level of academic effort so that they may do what is required of them as employees.

The perspectives of interns are not peculiar to medical education. The graduate student at a university must take courses, work on a thesis or dissertation, attend to teaching or research duties he may have, and prepare for comprehensive examinations. Though faculty consider the examinations an intellectual challenge requiring intense preparation, students consider preparation of the sort expected too much to do. They reject the faculty idea that the examination is an intellectual challenge and approach it as a hurdle rather than as an educational experience. Students, therefore, evolve perspectives that will result in knowledge necessary to pass the examinations and not a plan to obtain an understanding or add to knowledge of their subject.[4] The situation is such that students cannot do all they have

4. The problems faced by graduate students is discussed in David Mechanic, *Students Under Stress* (New York, Free Press, 1962). A significant point of Mechanic's discussion is that graduate students have a great deal to do but time is limited and every student must solve the

to do, and their perspective reflects a reduced level of academic effort that is, if not encouraged, tolerated by the faculty.

The physicians of the Harvard Medical Unit, in much the same way that faculties do, tolerate a reduced level of effort on some activities to make it possible for interns to cope with the demands of their work. A maximum effort—an effort to "do it all"—might incapacitate interns and reduce their value as a part of the hospital's labor force. Effort expended on academic activities would certainly require a reduction of effort directed toward patient care. Physicians therefore tolerate a reduced acadmic effort, permitting interns to adopt a perspective that does not conflict with the hospital's function as a service facility rather than an educational institution. The way interns coordinate learning and work is exactly what is necessary to facilitate the hospital's operations and maintain the Unit as a part of the hospital and a viable segment of the medical elite.

---

problem of allocating time and effort in an advantageous way. The implication of his discussion and of what I have said is that those responsible for educational programs establish requirements that are impractical, and the perspectives of interns and students reflect the impracticality of educational requirements by legitimizing reduced levels and altered directions of effort.

9. Is an Elite Internship Different?

INTERNS repeatedly told me that things were different at other hospitals. "Interns at other hospitals don't have the problems we do, and don't have to do as much as we do," Harvard interns told me. Since I had no comparative data on other hospitals, I arranged to spend a few weeks at a general hospital in a Boston suburb. My reason for doing so was to determine if, in fact, other internships were so different from the elite training I observed.

My first visit to the suburban hospital startled me after my year at BCH. This hospital was not old nor in obvious need of repair. The equipment was modern. There were many nurses on the wards. The first day I spent with an intern further convinced me that this was certainly a different medical setting. When I learned that interns had no trouble getting clean uniforms, I recalled all the times I had wandered around Boston City Hospital with interns in search of laundry. When I asked the intern how much laboratory work he had to do, he said, "I don't do any, because the lab people do everything for me."

When we visited a patient, we entered a room in which there were only four patients, but five nurses. Also, the intern I was with left the hospital to have lunch with his family.

My first few days at the general hospital consisted almost entirely in making these sorts of comparisons. As I spent more time with the interns, however, I found that they were doing very many of the same things as interns on the Harvard Medical Services. The settings were different, but I actually saw no startling differences in the work.

Like the Harvard internship at BCH, this program emphasized learning by doing. Interns at both hospitals were expected to make work rounds with a resident twice daily, were responsible for working up patients, and were charged with day-to-day patient care. At both hospitals interns rotated through the outpatient department, the admitting floor, and the emergency ward.

Since the data I had collected by participant observation did not tell me whether there were real differences between the two groups, I decided to make more precise measures. Therefore I conducted a time study of the activity of three interns randomly selected from each group. The following data and interpretations are based on the results of that study.

I recruited and trained a number of my students to record intern activity. Three of these were in the Graduate Training Program in the Social Organization of Medical Care. All had some experience in a variety of medical settings. The training, which took place a few weeks before they went into the field to collect data, stressed accuracy of recording and agreement on the kinds of tasks to be assigned to each category of activity. Each student observed five days of activity by a different intern at each hospital, recording the time interns spent on each kind of activity.

Other studies have determined that a period of five consecutive days affords a reliable sample of work.[1] Since weekends

1. The observation procedures were similar to those suggested by Margaret G. Arnstein, *How to Study Nursing Activities in a Patient Unit* (Washington, D.C., U.S. Government Printing Office, 1954). I had previously employed similar procedures. See Stephen J. Miller and W. D. Bryant, *A Division of Nursing Labor* (Kansas City, Mo., Smith Grieves Co., 1965).

were in no way special at either hospital, the data are based on the period from Monday through Friday. The observers' task was to record what each intern was doing at thirty-minute intervals during the day, in terms of specific categories of activity. They also wrote brief descriptions of the activity. For each intern studied, a new series of observations was started every thirty minutes, so that half of each working hour was classified according to the categories of activity. On the first day observations started at 8:00 A.M. and progressed from 9:00 A.M., 10:00 A.M., and so on. On the next day they started at 8:30 A.M. and continued at 9:30 A.M., 10:30 A.M., and so on. If there was some regularly scheduled activity, such as a conference, observers watched interns only if they did not attend. Observers were rotated among interns so that each made observations of different interns at different times of the day.

The data represent the work of a forty-hour week at each hospital, excluding time spent on work rounds, visiting rounds, and other scheduled activity. The percentage of time interns spent in scheduled activities is presented in Figure 9.1. This is not to say that interns spend their time this way every single day, but on an average day interns at both hospitals spent approximately 40 to 50 per cent of their time making work rounds or attending some scheduled activity. The rest of their time, however, had to be further defined and analyzed before differences could be discerned between the groups.

The data in Figure 9.1 represent only the interns' work between 8:30 A.M. and 5:00 P.M. at the general hospital, and 8:00 A.M. and 5:00 P.M. at Boston City Hospital. Evening and night work are omitted. The data cover the activity of interns when they are on their own approximately 50 per cent of the time. According to plan, a different three and one-half hours of free time was sampled each day. Excluding regular activities, interns at the general hospital had 1,170 minutes and those at BCH 1,350 minutes of free time. The schedule for observations, if followed exactly, would have resulted in our observing all the free time of interns at the general hospital and sampling 75 per cent of that of BCH interns. It was not possible, however, to follow the schedule exactly, because interns were not always available when we wanted them, took ill, or left the hospital early. In the five days of observation, we were able to sample 82 per cent of the free time of interns at the general hospital. We also adjusted the schedule to permit observation of interns who started work early, which resulted in an 88 per cent sample of the free time of interns at BCH.[2]

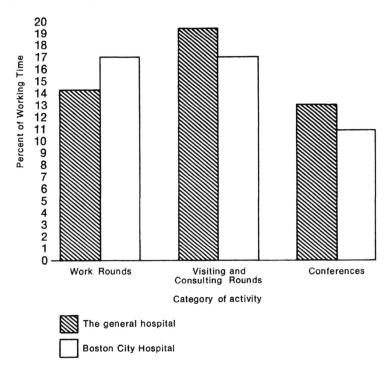

Figure 9.1. Comparison between the Daily Activity of Interns at the General Hospital and That of Interns at Boston City Hospital

2. The intern's free time was computed as the amount of time he spent at the hospital, less the time he participated in scheduled activity. Interns spent, on the average, 2,250 minutes per week at the general hospital, of which 1,080 minutes were scheduled. Of the remaining 1,170 minutes, 955, or 82 per cent, were observed and classified according to categories of activities. Interns spent 2,550 minutes at Boston City Hospital, 1,200 scheduled. Of the remaining 1,350 minutes, 1,185, or 88 per cent, were observed and classified. The data reported in this chapter were computed from these samples of activity.

When the data were analyzed, it was obvious that the three observers did not always agree on the category to which each task should be assigned. The fact that observers were required to describe each task they observed made it possible to correct such discrepancies. When there was an inconsistency of this sort, I assigned the task to a category. Since interns sometimes performed several tasks simultaneously, it was not always possible to determine to the minute how much time they spent on each.

The observations were limited to certain hours because interns were most accessible at those times. The comparison between groups, therefore, is obviously limited to their daytime activities. My students missed much of the flavor of the work at both hospitals because, as observers, they had the specific task of recording activity. They did not spend time with interns unless they were observing. The data presented in Figure 9. 1 are also somewhat misleading. For example, they indicate that the two groups of interns spent approximately the same amount of time in academic activity. We know, though, that interns at BCH often decide to miss a conference in order to gain more time for other kinds of activity. Interns at the general hospital did the same when they were on ward rather than on private services.

The following comments by an intern illustrate the difference between the ward and private services:

> I have a lot of time to read on the private service, and I can attend all the conferences and lectures. If I was still on service, I wouldn't be at today's conference. You have a lot more to do on service. The patients are sicker, too. Now, on the private services, I admit them and it's up to their doctors to take care of them. I have to worry about this guy with the drips, but private patients aren't my worry. On the service wards you have a lot of responsibility, but you don't have it on the private side. [March 8, 1965]

Thus we see that, contrary to Figure 9.1, interns at the general hospital spend much more time on academic activity when they are assigned to the private services.

Though the general hospital used private as well as ward patients for teaching purposes, we observed the interns there only on the wards. The reason for this is, of course, that the BCH interns had no experience comparable to work on the private services.

What follows is a discussion of only "direct patient care" and "other" activity; that is, a more detailed discussion of activities when interns are not engaged in academic activity. For discussion I present four categories of work: (1) management of the medical setting; (2) exchange of information; (3) direct patient care; and (4) supplementary patient care. Each category is defined and discussed separately.

MANAGEMENT OF THE MEDICAL SETTING

Interns at both hospitals engaged in activities that are not patient care per se, but arrangement for facilities or services that make it possible to take care of patients. These activities included obtaining necessary equipment, arranging for social services, collecting supplies, and similar tasks by which interns try to control the physical environment.

The observed management tasks may be further divided into five classes of activity:

1. *Communication* on the ward consisted almost entirely of informing nurses of the condition of equipment, hazardous spills or objects, and the need for supplies, as well as requesting specimens, equipment, and changes in the patient area and ward conditions. The purpose of other communication was to inform attending physicians of patient requests, or to notify hospital authorities of changes in a patient's condition. Interns would, for example, inform social service of an imminent discharge or arrange to remove a patient's name from the danger list to avoid administrative problems in discharging him.

2. *Telephoning* is simply another method of communication, but we report it separately because we could quite accurately measure the time spent in this way. Interns used the telephone to solicit consultation or to arrange for some other service for

a patient. The decision to consider time on the telephone a management task rather than some other kind of activity was arbitrary. Time on the telephone could also be considered exchange of information, but that category of activity had, by definition, been limited to discussion of the specific problems of particular patients.

3. *Locating equipment* refers not to requisitioning but to actually securing, conveying, and setting up equipment required for treatment or diagnosis. The category includes all tasks necessary to learn the location of equipment; travel time to get it and bring it to the ward; and returning it to its proper storage place.

4. *"Running around"* includes all the interns' efforts to expedite their work. This colloquialism focuses attention on a critical category of activity. Locating equipment is a part of it, but we reported separately the time spent in this way, since we could measure it very accurately. Running around includes going after patient records, taking specimens to the laboratory or picking up laboratory tests, making trips to other hospital departments to schedule services for patients—in other words, all the tasks we usually think are done by nonprofessional employees.

5. *Transporting patients* is really more running around, but again, since we could measure it accurately, we reported it separately. Interns bring patients from the admitting floor to the ward. When there are no porters available, they may themselves transport their patients to another hospital department. Such things as getting patients out of bed and sitting in chairs we recorded as direct patient care.

Figure 9.2 shows the percentage of their time interns at the two hospitals were observed to spend managing their respective medical settings. Although the data do reflect differences in activity, they are not presented as definitive profiles of how interns spend their time when managing their medical settings.

Interns at BCH spent approximately twice as much time managing the medical setting as interns at the general hospital. At the general hospital these activities cost the intern less than half an hour of his time each day, while at BCH an intern had to spend more than half again as much time in this way.

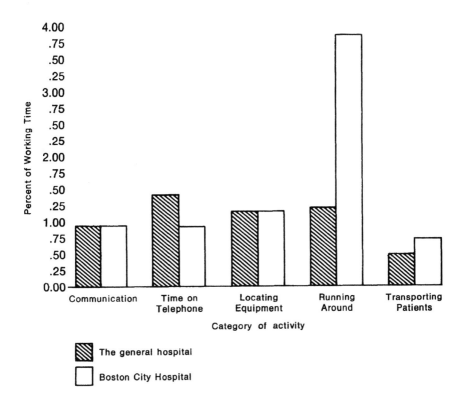

Figure 9.2. Comparison between the Percentage of Time Interns at the General Hospital and Interns at Boston City Hospital Spend on the Management of Their Medical Setting

Interns at the two hospitals spent the same amount of time in communication and locating equipment. It is important to note that this communication had to do directly with the management of the medical setting. There was, of course, a great deal more communication among hospital personnel, and much more time was spent on the telephone discussing patients and their problems. Interns at BCH had to spend a few more minutes each day transporting patients, but the difference between hospitals does not appear to be significant. The important difference was in the amount of time interns spent running around the hospital. Interns at BCH were observed to spend almost half an hour each day in this way, as compared to a few minutes at the general hospital. In other words, interns at Boston City Hospital do more for themselves to expedite their work. Most of what they do, however, is arranging for or obtaining the results of laboratory work.

A number of circumstances at Boston City Hospital may explain this difference in activity. First, the hospital is not adequately staffed. Second, patients here may be sicker than those at the general hospital. If this were so, interns would want information as quickly as possible, which could explain their efforts to speed up laboratory work. Another possibility that must not be overlooked is that interns at a university-affiliated hospital may order more laboratory work than interns at a general hospital. Administrators at BCH often complained that the Harvard interns ordered more laboratory work than necessary; they attributed this to what they called "the academic way of thinking." Interns at the general hospital, in fact, did no laboratory tests themselves, but we have no data on their actual use of the laboratories. Interns at BCH did spend 4 per cent of their time running around, compared to 1 per cent for interns at the general hospital.

Whatever the reasons, the fact remains that interns at Boston City Hospital spent significantly more time managing their medical setting than those in the comparison group. Allowing for the fact that medical records are harder to get at BCH, most of the variation can be accounted for by the amount of time Harvard interns spend arranging for or obtaining results from laboratories and the X-ray department.

EXCHANGE OF INFORMATION

Most people at a hospital need to know the conditions of and services required by the patients. The exchange of information among these people is what permits the organization of patient care. All tasks that informed medical, nursing, and other per-sonnel of a patient's condition were reported as exchange of information. The category was further broken down according to the type and purpose of the information exchanged.

The most obvious difference between the two hospitals in activity of this sort concerned the exchange of information for teaching purposes. Since there were no medical students at the general hospital, interns obviously spent no time talking with them. Interns at BCH, however, spent almost 5 per cent of their time instructing medical students or exchanging information relevant to patient care. The other categories of information exchange were applicable at both hospitals: (1) exchange pertinent to diagnosis, including the evaluation of laboratory results and discussions with consulting physicians; (2) exchange pertinent to the choice of a treatment plan, particularly information relevant to the choice of a medical procedure; (3) reporting a patient's condition to other physicians; and (4) informing nursing personnel of changes in a patient's condition or of new orders concerning medication or treatments. This includes verbal communication only, not charting or writing orders.

Figure 9.3 shows the amount of time interns at the two hospitals were observed to spend in information exchange. These data do not include information exchange at regularly scheduled meetings, such as visiting rounds, work rounds, or conferences. This category, like the others, covers only unscheduled time.

Harvard interns spent more time exchanging information than their general hospital counterparts. When the times are corrected to take into account the teaching function of the Harvard interns, however, the difference all but vanishes.

While the differences in time spent exchanging information may not be significant, there is no interesting difference in the kinds of information exchanged. Interns at the two hospitals spent almost the same amount of time conversing with nurses and discussing diagnosis and treatment, but those at BCH did spend much less time reporting the condition and progress of their patients to other physicians. The BCH interns reported to the residents, but those at the general hospital were more often questioned by visiting physicians. The residents at both hospitals were responsible for the administration of the wards, but interns at the general hospital appeared to defer more often to the visiting physician. Residents at the general hospital were, of

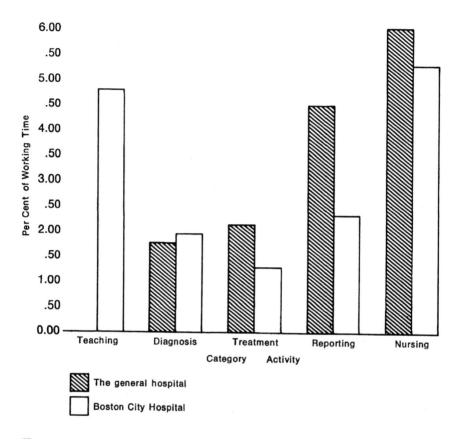

Figure 9.3 Comparison between the Percentage of Time Interns at the General Hospital and Interns at Boston City Hospital Spend on the Exchange of Information

course, active in discussion about diagnosis and treatment, but day-to-day patient care appeared to be more under the supervision of visiting physicians, who made many if not most of the medical decisions. At BCH the intern and his resident themselves made decisions concerning diagnosis and treatment, often without discussing them with the visiting or any other physician. Physicians apparently supervised patient care more actively at the general hospital, which could explain why interns spent so much of their time reporting to them. Interns at BCH spent much less of their time in this way, usually with a consulting rather than a visiting physician.

The data suggest that interns at the general hospital are closely supervised by staff physicians. Their medical responsibility is, in a sense, limited by the opinions of practicing physicians. Interns at BCH are limited less by the opinions of physicians than by those of residents, who are more like interns than like practicing physicians. The implications of such a difference for the experience of interns is an area that requires further study. The immediate implication, however, is that full-fledged physicians have less to say about medical care at Boston City Hospital than at the general hospital.

DAY-TO-DAY PATIENT CARE

This general type of activity was divided into two subcategories. *Direct patient care* includes tasks done in the presence of the patient—taking medical histories, doing physical examinations, and performing diagnostic or continuous procedures, as well as carrying out required treatments. *Supplementary patient care* included all tasks necessary for the preparation or delivery of direct patient care—things most often done in the laboratory or at the nursing station on the ward. Together direct and supplementary patient care make up the bulk of an intern's work at both hospitals.

Interns at both hospitals spent approximately the same amount of time on direct patient care. There were differences, however, in the amount of time devoted to particular tasks. The breakdown is presented in Figure 9.4.

Working up a patient consists of taking a medical history and doing a physical examination. Interns at the two hospitals did not work up patients in the same way. Those at the general hospital spent more time taking histories and less time on physical examinations than those at BCH. Since it was difficult to classify questions asked of patients when they were being examined, we made the distinction purely on the basis of chronology. The time reported on taking a history represents only

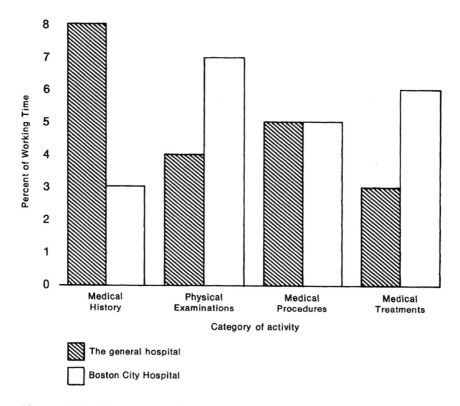

Figure 9.4. Comparison between the Percentage of Time Interns at the General Hospital and at Boston City Hospital Spend on Direct Patient Care

the time an intern spent questioning a patient before he began the actual physical examination, after which his time was recorded as examining, even though he continued to question the patient regarding complaints and symptoms.

The BCH interns spent significantly less time taking a history before they began a physical examination. This difference may be explained in part by differences in the two hospitals' patient populations. Patients at the general hospital are middle class, usually admitted by a family physician, while those at BCH are lower class, usually brought or coming to the hospital without having seen a physician. Many do not speak English; others may be senile or incoherent; still others simply do not communicate well, especially in medical terms. Thus the interns had to depend more on the results of their examinations.

Interns at the two hospitals were observed to spend the same amount of time in diagnostic procedures, including collecting and labeling specimens and positioning patients. The BCH interns, however, spent a good deal more of their time on such treatments as inhalation therapy, enemata, catheterizations, irrigations, dressings, and ambulation. They also spent more time checking to make sure that nurses were carrying out the ordered treatments. At the general hospital most of the treatments listed here were routinely delegated to nursing personnel. Much of this difference is, of course, attributable to the shortage of nurses at BCH.

Interns at the two hospitals also spent approximately the same amount of time on supplementary patient care, though again with differences in what they did. First, as we have seen, interns at the general hospital did no laboratory work. At BCH interns were required to do all routine analysis of blood and urine, as well as some cultures and other laboratory tests. Second, interns at the general hospital spent significantly more time than those at BCH in reading the medical literature. The data presented in Figure 9.5 would indicate that they do have time to read and still do their work, though they are on a service comparable to the Harvard Medical Services. Finally, interns at BCH spent more time charting and reading results of tests, observations, and notes about their patients. When questioned about this difference, one intern said, "You spend more time reading the charts because the residents write long notes, and you write long notes because the resident reads the charts." On the other hand, an intern at the general hospital said, "Everybody is writing in the charts. How much can you add to what the physician puts down or tells you to put down? I read the charts to bring myself up-to-date about patients after I have a day or two off." The patient charts at BCH appear to serve a purpose other than the intended one: They are a means

of communication and control between the intern and the resident. At the general hospital these are apparently achieved
through direct reports to physicians.

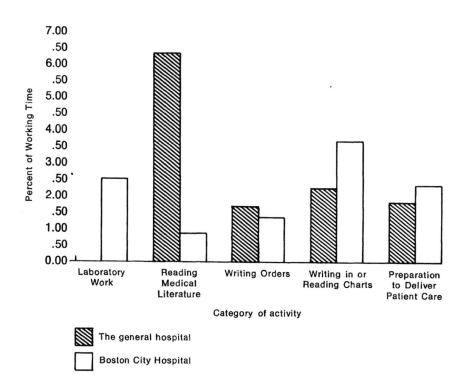

*Figure 9.5. Comparison between the Percentage of Times
Interns at the General Hospital and Interns at Boston City
Hospital Spend on Supplementary Patient Care*

Interns at Boston City Hospital were also observed to spend
more time preparing to give care to their patients. Since the
time required to get equipment and medications was sometimes
recorded here as well as under "locating equipment," it is impossible to say that there actually was a difference between the
two groups in this preparation time.

THE DIFFERENCE BETWEEN "GOOD" AND "THE BEST"

A cursory comparison of the activities of interns at the general hospital and those of Harvard interns at BCH would reveal no startling differences. They apparently spend the same relative amounts of time on many of the same kinds of activity. My time study of three randomly selected interns at each hospital does, however, indicate some important differences.

I have suggested before that serving an internship with an elite medical group is different from serving with a group that is merely good. The differences are not so much due to the nature of the work itself as to the purposes of the two groups of physicians conducting the training programs. The fact that the primary purpose of the Harvard Medical Unit is research, not teaching, means that staff physicians are too busy with their own investigations to spend much time teaching. This means, in turn, that interns are taught by residents instead of full-fledged physicians. The fact that BCH physicians delegated a great deal of their teaching responsibility was the most obvious difference between the two programs. Physicians at the general hospital were apparently more active teachers. A more subtle difference grows out of Harvard physicians' being less interested in routine patient care than physicians at the general hospital. Physicians at BCH delegated this responsibility to interns, assistant residents, and residents. At the general hospital the intern's experience is considerably different.

> I met Harrison on the private service and asked what he was going to do that afternoon. He said, "I have some procedures to do." I asked if these were on service or private patients. "They're things that the physicians want me to do for their patients." "Do you mean they're procedures they just left notes for you to do?" Harrison nodded and said, "Yes, they're things they want done for their patients here and some things I have to do on the ward side. I don't always see them, so they just write down what they want me to do."
>
> I asked him if he had any say in what was done for the patients. He said, "I can get in touch with the patient's doctor,

but I don't usually do that. I don't get a great deal of responsibility for what's done on the private side. That's why I go over to the other side. I go over there because I get a lot of teaching over there." I remarked that it looked like he had a great deal of free time on the private side. "Yes, on this side you get a chance to read and do a lot of other things. You don't have these chances on the other side." I asked why that was so. "With the ward patients, you have some responsibility. You have to decide what needs to be done and see that it gets done. I guess, in a way, you're more the doctor over there. Over here, the patients have their own doctors."

We started to walk off when he stopped as if he remembered something and returned to one of the rooms. I waited for him. When he returned he said, "There was a patient I had to see. There were just one or two things her doctor wanted to know, and he asked me to find out for him. She's just in for a general looking-over, and there were some things her doctor wanted to be sure of. They keep an eye on what you're doing for their patients." [March 16, 1965]

An intern at the general hospital is less his own man than the Harvard intern. Physicians tell him most of what he must do; the intern at BCH is responsible for patient care all year.

Interns at the general hospital spent a great deal more time with the physicians assigned to the service. The physicians assigned to teach also exercised their responsibility for patient care. They required interns to report and consult with them, even on ward services (see Figure 9.3). There is no doubt that interns at the two hospitals received advice and direction regarding patient care from two different sources. The Harvard interns were supervised and taught by residents, not by physicians. The Harvard physicians discovered that by delegating responsibility they were able to control the situation without great expense of time and effort. They maintained the viability of their medical services by delegating authority to interns, rather than by exercising it as the general hospital physicians did. By maximizing the interns' responsibility, the Harvard Medical Unit could provide patient care without interfering with its essential purpose, research.

When considering the social organization of the Harvard

Medical Unit, one cannot help being impressed by the way it operates. First, there is the way students, interns, and residents are used to prepare one another for the work they have to do if the organization is to persist. The absence of a similar process of succession at the general hospital requires that interns learn the ropes from physicians. These physicians obviously must spend more time with interns, though it is also for opportunity to control what interns will do. Then there is the delegation of responsibility to young men who are only too anxious to have it. The fact that they have the responsibility, however, also requires the BCH interns to spend more of their time managing the medical setting. Medical school has prepared most interns to manage their patients medically, but Harvard interns are called on to develop other managerial skills. The Harvard interns spend significantly more of their time managing their medical setting and doing teaching and laboratory work usually handled by physicians or technicians at general hospitals. This is, of course, a saving of time by Harvard physicians. Interns at the general hospital spend much less of their time in this way. They spend almost half of their time in academic activity, at which the Harvard interns spend a quarter of their time. These differences may also be attributed to the differential responsibility delegated to the interns. Those who are more preoccupied with patient care have less time to read. The way in which the Harvard Medical Unit maintains itself as an elite segment may, some would say, conflict with the educational goals of interns. By making so much of the work of an internship managerial, the Harvard physicians preclude the interns' extensive participation in academic activity. Many physicians would argue, however, that an internship of this sort is more valuable because of the responsibility it offers. This, of course, results in practical experience, which is the purpose of an internship. If the idea of responsibility, which is so highly valued in medical education, is taken as the criterion, then interns at the general hospital may have a less valuable experience than those at Boston City Hospital.

The responsibility we are talking about is not only for diagnosis and treatment, but also for the management of the medical setting. The experience of the Harvard interns may not be necessary to prepare young men for careers in medicine. There may also be, as interns apparently conclude, such a thing as too much responsibility. The Harvard internship program does apparently serve the straightforward purpose of providing the first responsibility young men have for the welfare of patients. It also serves, however, to reduce teaching demands on Harvard physicians and allows them to divest themselves of routine patient care so they can do research.

Interns at both hospitals had similar jobs to do; they had the responsibility for providing patient care. The significant difference was the way in which their efforts were used by other physicians. Physicians at the community hospital acted to control interns assisting them, for purposes of patient care. Interns at the community hospital served the purpose of practicing physicians by caring for patients and thereby facilitating the operation of that hospital and assisting physicians with their medical practices. The Harvard interns did the same; that is, facilitated the operation of the hospital. More than that, however, they also relieved Harvard physicians of a responsibility which would curtail other activities and thereby assisted them with their clinical investigations. Interns were exploited at both hospitals but for different purposes. The difference, then, was not what they did but which purpose they served. At Boston City Hospital the exploitation of interns served the purpose of the medical elite as well as the straightforward purpose of trained young physicians.

10. Conclusion

SOCIOLOGISTS interested in medical education have conducted much research and reported many findings. The literature is replete with differences of sociological opinion, indicative of the diverse theoretical analyses of medical education. A review of that literature has been compiled and published.[1] The purpose of this chapter is not to further review the literature but to discuss the particular significance of the present study. Although sociologists have conducted much research, the focus of most sociological studies has been the medical school. Programs of graduate medical education have not received sufficient attention; the internship has been considered only incidentally, though it is a mandatory year of medical education.[2] My study

1. See Samuel W. Bloom, "The Sociology of Medical Education," *Milbank Memorial Fund Quarterly*, 43, 2 (April, 1965), pp. 174–184.
2. Sociologists at Columbia University have been among the few concerned with the internship, and a report of those studies is soon to be published by Harvard University.

has provided data regarding this year, and thus far has been highly descriptive. In conclusion it is necessary to indicate its place within the context of sociology, and elaborate the implications of the study.

Medical education consists of stages, each assumed to impart knowledge and perfect skills characteristic of physicians. The young men and women who make the grade at college present themselves and their records to the committees which admit or refuse to admit them to medical schools. If they are admitted, they are in the initial stage of medical education, or the preclinical years. Those admitted who make the grade during the first years and subsequent clinical years of medical school are permitted to go on to the next stage, the internship. Medical school graduates must, in fact, serve internships to qualify as practicing physicians, since an internship is considered the final stage of education before the independent practice of medicine. Medical educators conceptualize the stages as logically related educational experiences: Medical schools, during the preclinical years, impart the knowledge basic to medicine; the clinical years of school and the internship add knowledge, perfect skills, and introduce fledgling physicians to full-fledged physicians who exhibit in their work the practices of acceptable physicians. Medical education, therefore, consists of stages which in turn consist of educational experiences that facilitate the progressive acquisition of a collectivity of characteristics required of persons permitted to practice medicine.

Sociology has alternated between analyses of medical education that emphasize the medical educators' conceptualization, and analyses that concede it is a likely explanation but an unnecessary emphasis for sociological explanation of the stages of medical education. Sociological analyses of medical schools emphasizing acquisition of "professional" characteristics are exemplified by studies by the Bureau of Applied Research at Columbia University.[3] Those studies assumed that medical students were learning the role of a physician by gradually acquiring the collectivity of characteristics required of physicians. An

3. See Robert K. Merton, George Reader, and Patricia L. Kendall, *The Student Physician* (Cambridge, Harvard University Press, 1957).

example of an alternate analysis is the study of the University of Kansas.[4] That study assumed the school to be a stage of medical education posing specific and immediate problems, not necessarily related to the realities of medical practice, which had to be resolved before students could go on to meet subsequent requirements for the attainment of the status "physician." The demands of the school required that they learn. the role of "student," not "physician," and it turned their attention to the immediate business of getting through medical school.

The two approaches to medical education that have been briefly noted have both contributed to the explanation of medical education. If sociologists accept as their assumption the medical educator's conceptualization, then it is logical to analyze the internship as the stage which adds the final characteristics necessary for the acceptable practice of medicine.

There is evidence, however, that the actual practice of medicine is as much the result of realities for which physicians are not prepared as of their education.[5] This is not to say that medical education does not impart knowledge and perfect skills crucial for the acceptable practice of medicine. Rather it is to say that the acquired knowledge and perfected skill will be applied in situations which are difficult to duplicate in existing training settings. The evidence being what it is, sociologists are paying less attention to the future implications of any particular stage of medical education and more attention to the immediate problems of trainees during their training. My study of a Harvard internship, for that reason, is aligned with the study of the University of Kansas, and so identifiable by the assumption

4. See Howard S. Becker, Blanche Geer, Everett C. Hughes, and Anselm L. Strauss, *Boys in White* (Chicago, University of Chicago Press, 1961).

5. See, among others, Melvin Seeman and John W. Evans, "Stratification and Hospital Care: The Performance of the Medical Intern," *American Sociological Review*, 26 (February, 1961), pp. 67–80; George E. Miller, ed., *Teaching and Learning in Medical School* (Cambridge, Harvard University Press, 1961); Osler L. Peterson and others, *An Analytical Study of North Carolina General Practice* (Evanston, Ill., Association of American Medical Colleges, 1956); and Eliot Friedson, "The Organization of Professional Behavior," a paper read at the annual meeting of the American Sociological Association at Montreal, 1964.

underlying the analysis presented in preceding chapters: that the internship is an apprenticeship conducted in the hospital, an organization which poses specific problems that must be resolved by interns before they are permitted to practice medicine or go on to further training for a variety of careers in the medical profession.

Though I have reported a study of medical education, my concern is with the more general phenomenon of professional education and its processes as they exist in training settings. The internship is, of course, a program of instruction and supervised practice that provides knowledge of the basic sciences and their application in the diagnoses and treatment of disease. An internship as I have described it in preceding chapters is more than that; it is an apprenticeship of sorts and a way for physicians to recruit colleagues and successors. I have described an educational program that assures a segment of a profession suitable recruits in sufficient numbers for the careers it advocates, and discussed the training that prepares these recruits for those and other careers.

Many professions require the equivalent of an apprenticeship before inducting new members and according the status of professional. Social work, for example, requires that all candidates for its careers serve in one or another social service agency, under the supervision of practicing social workers, before awarding degrees and certifying them as professionals. There is not, however, a great deal of data available, and until studies are conducted it is permissible to assume that the apprenticeships of the other professions are much like the internships of the medical profession. Further, it may be assumed that the segments of other professions act in ways similar to those of the medical profession. The assumption is logical, since medicine has served as the prototype for the professions and, for that reason, what has been reported is relevant for the sociology of professions as well as for the sociology of medical education.

All people spend a part of their lives in organizations whose explicit purpose is to educate them. There are public and private schools which provide basic education; advanced education takes place in colleges, and specialized education in graduate and professional schools. Many people, however, spend a part of their lives in organizations whose explicit purpose is not to educate them but in which they are expected to learn and prepare for work. The least complicated example of such education is on-the-job training to do relatively menial work. A more complicated example is the internship or, more generally, professional apprenticeships. In them, people learn advanced techniques and perfect skills in organizations whose explicit purpose is not their education but the delivery of service. The internship is a program of the latter sort, and provides an opportunity to analyze the processes of professional education as they exist in organizations which are only incidentally concerned with education.

The internship is an apprenticeship for fledging physicians so they may learn medicine by actually providing patient care under the supervision of more experienced physicians. More than that, it takes place in an organization whose explicit purpose is not the education of physicians but the provision of patient care. The study reported here has described the experience of young men on the wards of Boston City Hospital. I have concluded that they choose a particular way of doing their work because their training is subservient to the primary purpose of the hospital. Stated another way: the primary purpose of the hospital determined the context of their training. This may well be the case for all candidates for the professions who are required to serve apprenticeships in the service organizations of their respective professions.

What, then, are the implications of the character of service organizations for the training of personnel for the professions? Many of its implications are common to all formal organizations: the table of organizations, staff and line relations, and decision making or authority. My emphasis, however, is on the characteristics common to organizations which as well as providing service, also attempt to prepare people for professional careers. The justification for this emphasis is simply that these characteristics are an important but little studied part of professional education.

The most common characteristic of organizations that exist to do things for or to the public is that they operate as systems for the delivery of service. The purpose of all such organizations is to provide services of a particular sort in the most feasible way. Service organizations are, of course, highly differentiated systems, with many purposes other than the delivery of service. Another of its purposes is often the training of people to perform the specialized tasks which are allocated to the different groups that comprise the organization. Many would argue that there is no better setting for the training of these people than the organizations in which they will eventually occupy positions and do their work. There is, however, a problem in doing so, and though I have alluded to it throughout my description of a medical internship, the problem must be reiterated because of its implications for all such training.

Service organizations are systems within which training takes place, and not systems whose explicit purpose is training. Organizations of this sort have evolved as delivery systems with little regard for the potential conflict between the work that must be done and what people must learn, and all work must be specifically and directly related to the providing of service. Work at the hospital as I have described it was often in conflict with lectures, conferences, and other activity unrelated to work. Work was not always consistent with the educational purposes of an internship, and interns had to be highly adaptable and imaginative to coordinate their efforts to learn with efforts to do their work. This is an implication of the character of service organizations, and apparently a particular problem with training that occurs within service organizations.

The approach I have taken in describing the internship studied is basically simple: Interns face a problematic situation, requiring them to determine how to satisfy the purpose of an internship and do the work which will serve the purpose of the hospital. The demands of work are, of course, an obstacle that must be overcome before interns resolve the problems inherent in their situation. They must learn where things and people are, the implications of rank and privilege, the expectations of those with whom they must work and who are permanent members of the organization. Further, they must learn what the rules are, which rules can or must be broken, which followed to the letter. The failure to learn these things necessary to do the work they are assigned may preclude learning anything else. They must, before they learn anything else, learn the ropes.

Organizations whose explicit purpose is education establish procedures to facilitate learning the ropes. Many provide orientation programs, tutors, or allow a period of time for the newcomer to adjust to the organization. The educational organizations are structured to facilitate such learning. Organizations that provide services and make use of trainees to do so cannot, however, interrupt the routine of work to facilitate learning by newcomers. There can be little doubt that organizations structured for other purposes make learning the ropes difficult and that trainees must be capable of considerable ingenuity in finding teachers.

Interns had to accumulate facts about the people with whom they had to work, and define for themselves what was appropriate in their situation. The processes by which interns and other trainees accumulate facts specific to a particular organization is seldom dignified with the label "learning." More often than not, this sort of learning is considered an adjustment to the organization expected of every newcomer. My description of the internship, however, implies that this process is more important than it is usually thought to be, and that the ability to learn the ropes is related to the successful completion of training. A knowledge of the ropes was critical for mastery of the situation by the new intern, and his subsequent success was dependent on the advantageous use of that knowledge. Success, in the case of the intern, entailed managerial skill which required a knowledge of the ropes. If there is a capacity for learning of this sort distinct from that for ordinary learning, as there may be, trainees may fail because they have not learned the ropes—a kind of learning seldom provided for in educational organizations, much less service organizations.

The ingenuity of interns in finding people to teach them the ropes supports my contention that this process is critical to the entire process of education; that is, interns know that failure to learn the ropes will make other kinds of learning impossible.

My data demonstrate that interns made use of any frequent social contact as an occasion for learning the ropes. If teaching physicians are not available, they turn to residents with only a year or two more experience than they themselves have; if residents are not available, they make use of students, ancillary personnel, and patients. They learn to tactfully exploit superiors and subordinates so that they may resolve their problematic situation.

The data also demonstrate that interns continue to tactfully exploit people at the hospital, and that this is a characteristic tactic of interns throughout their training. Though they may have solved the initial problem of learning the ropes, there are other problems still to be solved which require improvisation and diplomacy. There were, for example, many physicians who were potentially valuable consultants and teachers, but these physicians had their own work to do and resisted other demands for their time. Interns had much to gain by obtaining the assistance of more experienced physicians.

A persisting problem for interns was to obtain expert assistance, though doing so was to claim some of the time that experienced physicians would ordinarily spend on purposes other than teaching. A problem of this sort is not peculiar to interns or other kinds of trainees in service organizations. Graduate students face a similar problem: A newcomer to graduate school must in some way obtain the attention and assistance of the faculty. A study of graduate students suggests that those who have been in school for more than a year are more likely to obtain attention and assistance because they have demonstrated their potential and ability by withstanding the initial challenges.[6] There is the further suggestion that students survive by learning the ropes, and survival is an implicit claim for the attention and assistance of the faculty. There is an alternative explanation; that is, the student who learns the ropes not only survives but has knowledge which permits him not to claim but to negotiate for assistance. The newcomers who fail to learn the ropes are

6. See David Mechanic, *Students under Stress* (New York, Free Press, 1962), pp. 13–15.

more apt to receive attention than those who succeed.[7] The distinction in interpretation is subtle but, in my opinion, critical for an accurate understanding of the relationship between students and teachers, or apprentices and masters. The sociological import of the distinction is implicit in the following question: Is knowledge of the ropes simply a condition for survival which in turn serves as an implicit claim of trainees for expert assistance? Or is knowledge of the ropes not only a condition for survival but a prerequisite for negotiations by which trainees obtain assistance?

My data demonstrate that in a service organization knowledge of the ropes is a prerequisitive for negotiations by which interns obtain the expert opinion of consultants and teaching performances by knowledgeable physicians. The problem for the intern is, of course, greater than for the graduate student because the explicit purpose of graduate schools is educational; those organizations assign the task of instruction to specific people and delegate to them the responsibility for teaching. People who occupy positions in service organizations, on the other hand, are assigned numerous tasks or delegated responsibilities which leave little or no time for teaching. When this is the case, it is logical to conclude that trainees must know the ropes to determine what they have to exchange in return for the assistance and teaching they want. Teaching in service organizations must therefore be conceptualized as a process by which people negotiate the exchange of information and not as a right of students and an obligation of teachers.

Though students require only the assistance of their teachers, trainees in service organizations also require the assistance of other people with whom they must work. The assistance required, in the case of the intern, was provided by nursing and ancillary personnel. The hospital was, like other organizations, a hierarchy with rules defining the duties and responsibilities of its positions, and the positions affording differential status

7. Blanche Geer and others, "Learning the Ropes: Situational Learning in Four Occupational Training Programs," in Irwin Deutscher and Elizabeth J. Thompson, eds., *Among the People* (New York, Basic Books, 1968), p. 209.

and power. But rules were often vague, and not always binding, and could be interpreted or broken by nurses, technicians, and clerks who wished to expedite their work. Also, interns could not exercise the authority with which they were empowered by virtue of their positions.[8] The hospital could not be conceptualized as the highly structured organization it is usually thought to be, and the relationships of interns to its other personnel could not be explained in terms of official rules, job descriptions, or the assumed implications of status and power. My explanation of these relationships required that I conceptualize the hospital in terms of its informal rather than its formal structure; that is, as an organization in which interns, residents, nurses, and others were enmeshed in a process by which they negotiated courses of action that permitted them all to do the tasks they had to do.

Social relationships in service organizations must be conceptualized as processes by which personnel negotiate the exchange of information or assistance relevant to their respective work assignments. Interns were involved in numerous sets of exchange relationships, and many of those exchanges were necessary because the hospital had evolved a system for the delivery of patient care that was independent of its use for educational purposes. The interns employed the process of exchange to establish a network of relationships that served as a rudimentary social structure for the internship program. The structure for the internship was not so much prescribed by the hospital's normative patterns as it was negotiated between interns and residents, nurses, technicians, and all other personnel at the hospital. The implication is that all trainees serving apprenticeships may have to negotiate satisfactory relationships with more permanent personnel, and that the relationships are not idiosyncratic but the consistent result of social exchanges that are characteristic of service organizations.

When all else is said, the trainee in service organizations is still required to do his assigned work. The work of an internship has been described and I have documented how interns deter-

---

8. The reasons were discussed in preceding chapters; see also, David Mechanic, "Sources of Power of Lower Participants," *Administrative Science Quarterly*, VII (1962), pp. 349–364.

mined a level of effort and decided which activities they would direct that effort toward during the year. More could be said about the kinds of work interns did, but the actual work to be done differs from one hospital to another. Since my purpose is to elaborate only what service organizations have in common as training settings, it is sufficient to say that the level and direction of effort finally adopted by interns coincided with the purpose of a hospital as a service rather than an educational organization.

A particular implication of the observed manner in which interns determined a level and direction of effort is that trainees do not react idiosyncratically to their situation, nor do they always act in accord with the purposes of their training. A particular training program may affect individual trainees in a variety of ways, but each chooses a course of action similar to that of others sharing his situation. Interns had to select among many kinds of activities, deciding which required most of their effort and which required little or no effort at all. The fact that all interns decided to devote most of their effort to activities in keeping with the purposes of the hospital as a service organization implies a collective definition of that situation and a response that is considered logical given the realities of their immediate situation. The obvious conclusion is that the actions of trainees is as much a result of distinctive character of organizations in which they are trained as it is of individual differences or the sequence of study and work laid down for trainees. The necessity for social exchanges that permit other employees to encourage trainees to adopt certain courses of action is one such characteristic of service organizations.

A final characteristic that should be noted is that organizations whose purpose is service do not elaborate criteria for the success or failure of those who are brought into those organizations for the purposes of training. The criteria for success as an intern were obscure, and those in authority made no standard available by which an appropriate course of action could be determined. Interns could only evaluate themselves by comparing their activities to those of other interns. The only obvious indication of success was an ability to do the work assigned them, and interns could only compare themselves to other interns in terms of mastery of that work.

The internship as I have described it facilitates a collective definition of the situation emphasizing the importance of work, and a response requiring interns to devote most if not all their effort to doing that work. Thus interns come to the conclusion that what is most important for them to do is provide patient care. To do so, they divert effort from more academic pursuits —a decision which is eminently more logical than an effort to do all that is expected of them, because they are expected to do an impossible job: to care for patients and at the same time to attend lectures, conferences, meetings, and read the medical literature. Interns adopt the level and direction of effort they do partly because they find it virtually impossible under the circumstances to follow exactly the sequence of academic and service activities laid down by physicians planning their training.

Although the internship is an impossble job and interns must choose to provide patient care at the expense of academic pursuits, it could be argued that internships are viable stages of medical education because that is, in fact, their purpose. The original purpose of an internship was to provide fledging physicians with their first clinical experience and supervised responsibility for patients. A limited practice of this sort was to be a prelude to the independent practice of medicine. Today, however, the internship is not the first clinical experience; students serve clinical clerkships at hospitals and obtain much experience during the last two years of medical school. Also, an internship is not the final stage of a medical education. The typical medical career is now a specialty, which requires that education be continued by serving residencies. Though the original purpose of an internship no longer obtains, internships continue to be required and they persist as the apprenticeships of the medical profession.[9]

9. "A year is too much," interns have told me. "You can learn what there is to know in six months, and after that it's just going through the motions of patient care and may not be worth the time." A study conducted by the Bureau of Applied Social Research of Columbia University, reported by Patricia Kendall, indicates that only 25 per cent

I do not suggest that the internship does not improve clinical judgment, an important characteristic of physicians. The clinical competence of the interns I observed did improve (see Appendix I). What I suggest is that there must be some reason other than their original purpose for internships persisting as a mandatory stage of medical education. The most obvious reason is that hospitals need medical staffs, and interns occupy staff positions that must be filled if hospitals are to provide patient care. There is, however, another reason, and that is the structure of the medical profession.

The medical profession is not homogeneous, but an amalgamation of many groups of physicians. The members of one group do not always agree with the members of other groups on what is the essential purpose of medicine. There exists a diversity of purpose and differences of opinion concerning the relative value of the kinds of work physicians do or should be doing in our society. The differences that exist between groups of practitioners and academic groups exemplify the diversity. No collectivity of characteristics is shared by these physicians because they differentially value the work medicine claims as its own, and each group is characterized by special interests and commitment to a unique purpose.

The heterogeneity of medicine precludes conceptualization of internships as educational experiences which inculcate the characteristics stipulated for and common to all physicians. It is not possible for any profession whose members do not agree among themselves to present candidates for its career models who exhibit interests and a commitment that is commonly accepted, nor is it possible to stipulate all the characteristics of an acceptable professional. The internship, therefore, must be considered a mechanism employed by each group of physicians to introduce candidates for medical careers to models that are symbolic of the specific interests and commitments it values.

My description of a Harvard internship documents how candi-

---

of interns and residents considered what they were learning to be worth the time they spent caring for patients. See *The Graduate Education of Physicians* (Chicago, American Medical Association, 1966), p. 59.

dates for medical careers were recruited by one group of physicians. The purpose of that internship was not only to recruit and train candidates, but also to introduce potential colleagues and successors to models who exhibit the interest and commitment that is the core of careers in academic medicine. I have attempted to clarify how medical school graduates made their way to and took the first step on the ladder of these elite careers of the medical profession. Again, there is not a great deal of data available and therefore the implications of what I observed may also be applicable to the elite careers of other professions.

The internship is a mandatory stage of medical education. More than that it is apparently a process by which candidates for medical careers are recruited, trained, and distributed among the many groups of the medical profession. A logical assumption would be that the internships controlled by a specific group of physicians would be planned to prepare recruits for the particular career that the group advocates. This was not, however, the case in the Harvard internship I observed, though the Second and Fourth Medical Services at Boston City Hospital are noted for producing academic physicians.

Medical students chose to serve a Harvard internship because they sought careers as specialists, scientists, teachers, or of some combination of academic duties and specialty practice. A student choosing to serve this or another university-affiliated internship was announcing his candidacy for those kinds of careers. The subsequent careers of those who had served this particular internship demonstrate that those were, in fact, the kinds of careers likely to be had by the interns I observed at Boston City Hospital. My observations, however, demonstrate that the internship does not prepare interns particularly well for those careers. This is not to say that interns do not add to their knowledge of medicine, nor that they do not perfect medical technique. It is to say that much of what interns do is not pertinent or related to the realities of the kinds of careers they seek and which are advocated by Harvard physicians.

The implication of my observations is that the activities laid down for Harvard interns may be less important as educational activities than they are as a condition for access to elite careers.

No matter what interns may learn or which skills they perfect, sociologically this particular internship was a stage of medical education posing immediate problems, not necessarily related to the realities of future careers, which had to be successfully completed before interns could go on to meet the subsequent requirements for attainment of careers as specialists, scientists, educators, or some combination of one or another of those activities in the medical profession.

A further implication is that professional training must be so, or it would preclude the recruitment of uncommitted candidates for medical careers. My contention is that the drifter, the uncommitted candidate, is more common among professional trainees than is usually assumed. If drift is characteristic of trainees, how successful would recruitment be for programs that prepared trainees for specific careers? A training program that reduced career alternatives by not allowing trainees to remain uncommitted would reduce its pool of candidates and make it difficult to recruit colleagues and successors to the professionals who sponsor the training.

A significant reason for the success of elite internships is that they do allow interns to remain uncommitted. They may go on to a career in teaching and research; they may go into private practice; they may go on to a career in administration, planning, or the organization of medical care. All alternatives are open to them because they are not prepared for a specific career, but they are on the route that could lead to a career in academic medicine.

What I have said so far may appear contrary to what would be expected in this age of specialization. More often than not it is thought important for those who wish to specialize to commit themselves early in their careers. The increased knowledge and advanced technology of most professionals require many years of study and more years of advanced training. On the other hand, the professionals have assumed more and more of the responsibility for operating service organizations. The uncommitted candidate is an ideal person to perform the more menial and less complex tasks that need to be done, and educators who conduct programs in service organizations may for that reason tolerate drift during training.[10]

The internship is an excellent example; that is, interns, no matter what their reasons, perform the routine tasks of patient care and, by so doing, permit the specialists to devote most of their effort to their own work. The work of the medical elite is research, but they must provide service or the hospital will be lost to them as a clinical setting. The hospital is important because the elite requires its facilities and patient population for its research programs. But, since the actual operation of a hospital interferes with research, the elite can maintain itself by recruiting interns to provide routine patient care and residents to administer the wards.

Internships thus serve too important a function to be eliminated, though they no longer serve their original purpose. The internship now is the means of staffing research and teaching hospitals, and medical students must be recruited in sufficient numbers to provide patient care. If the Harvard Medical Unit did require that its interns be committed to elite careers it would recruit only students with elite aspirations. But the aspirations of many students are vague, and not every candidate for a medical career knows even by the time he is a senior resident what he wants as a medical career. So the Harvard Medical Unit must recruit drifters as well as students committed to the careers its physicians advocate for its staff at Boston City Hospital.

The graduates of almost any medical school could serve an elite internship; that is, they could do the work of an internship. But would the graduates of any medical school also be candidates for careers as specialists, teachers, and scientists? Many would not; they are committed to a career of general practice and that is not one of the careers advocated by the physicians of the Harvard Medical Unit. Such candidates would best ad-

10. A phenomenon that was also observed in social work; see Harvey W. Feldman and Stephen J. Miller, "The Implications of Professional Education for Careers in Public Assistance," a paper prepared for the American Public Welfare Association (Boston), September 5, 1968.

vance their careers by serving, for example, rotating internships at community hospitals. The continued existence of the Harvard Medical Unit depends on recruitment of medical school graduates who are not only willing and able to do the work of an internship, but who are also at least potential candidates for careers as scientists and teachers of medicine.

The recruitment of trainees by elite segments of professions is complicated because there is a need not only for manpower to staff the service organizations, but also for manpower with the potential to eventually collaborate with and replace the members of those segments[11] In order to survive, the elite segment must have new members; that cannot be left to chance alone, so segments of professions establish processes to recruit candidates who can do the work that must be done and who are also suitable candidates for careers of the elite.

The Harvard Medical Unit illustrates this feature of the elite. Though the work of an internship does not require interns to be of the highest caliber, the fact that they are potential colleagues and successors makes it imperative to recruit outstanding medical school graduates.

What I have attempted to do in this chapter is to elaborate the implications of what I observed for an understanding of professional training as it occurs in organizations whose explicit purpose is not education but the delivery of services. I have discussed some generalizations pertinent to an understanding of how a stage of professional education—the internship, or more generally, apprenticeships—are used by professional elites. Finally, I will briefly describe what is, in my opinion, the future of the medical elite.

A decade or more ago, a study of my sort would have elabo-

---

11. The elite internship serves all the purposes I discuss; those are: to provide fledgling-physicians with experience; to provide hospital staff who can deliver patient care; and to provide the medical elite with new members. The Harvard internship I observed served these purposes but the fact that it does may not be part of any explicit strategy of the medical elite. The Victorian public school is an example of an elite institution that served purposes which were not consciously intended. See Rupert Wilkinson, *Gentlemanly Power: British Leadership and the Public School Tradition* (London: Oxford University Press, 1964).

rated the principles of elite medical education. My description could well have served as a model for other medical schools attempting to establish themselves as quality institutions. What I observed obviously did interest many young physicians in the practice of elite medicine. The Harvard internships do produce physicians who practice a very necessary kind of medicine, one that has advanced medical knowledge and brought many diseases under control. But the practice of medicine is changing, and I think it is less valuable to discuss what has been than what will be.

The 1960's have seen the emergence of a new understanding of the practice of medicine. Medicine of this era is characterized by concern with chronic rather than episodic, acute disease; with the quality of medical care; with the coordination of medical services; and with the interrelation of education, health, and welfare.[12] Medicine is not always responsive to the demands of the public it serves, but the public of today is better informed and its demands cannot be ignored. More people than ever before are over 65, and they are demanding continuing and comprehensive care. Others are demanding and able to meet the cost of regular, preventive, comprehensive care. Prepayment plans and health insurance programs have made this possible. The response to these public demands is changing the medical profession.

Many developments outside the medical profession are influencing its practices. Physicians are concerned that new government funding policies may reduce the amount of money available for the support of basic medical research.[13] The Office of Economic Opportunity, which was established to conduct the War on Poverty, has financed community health centers, a departure from the traditional delivery of medical care. Made aware of the problems of the poor and the rising cost of health services, Congress had made money available for innovative systems of

12. William P. Shepard and James G. Eoney, Jr., "The Teaching of Preventive Medicine in the United States," *Milbank Memorial Fund Quarterly*, XLII, 4 (October, 1964).

13. "Is Basic Research Threatened" *Medical World News*, 7, 45 (December 2, 1966), pp. 108–119.

getting medical care to the people who need it. Medical care in the future will not be the exclusive responsibility of hospitals. There are now and will be more facilities that provide regular care to ambulatory patients and, when necessary, special care. Many new service organizations are emerging, as the university hospital and its services did in an earlier period.

Medical education is also being evaluated, and efforts are under way to implement changes in keeping with the new understanding of medicine. Medical schools are attempting to involve students, interns, and residents with patient's economic and social problems as well as their physical problems. The Citizens Commission of Graduate Medical Education has already recommended that training programs should emphasize continuing, preventive, comprehensive care. It further suggests that graduate education not be limited to the university hospital service, but that part of the time be spent in a comprehensive, continuing care service.

The physicians at medical schools and university-affiliated hospitals have been the elite of American medicine, but reputation and power shift as conditions change, and conditions are changing. The medical elite, therefore, faces a future of change and can no longer be committed only to the university type of medical service emphasizing research and the management of acute, episodic disease. The concept of continuing and comprehensive medical care is gaining more and more advocates. The medical elite may have changes forced on them, or they may guide the future direction of medicine and its practices in society.

As a sociologist, I have described the medical elite as it now exists. A new era is upon the medical profession. If the medical elite does not change its practices, it faces a future of diminishing influence. On the other hand, the medical elite could change and take the lead in implementing the new understanding of medicine. My responsibility as a sociologist is to clarify the alternatives and to indicate which are likely to obtain in our society. My hypothesis is that the medical elite will survive, though survival will require a change in the opinion of some members concerning the purpose of medicine.

My hypothesis is based on data obtained subsequent to the study. Though the data are not conclusive, they indicate that the elite will change because of efforts from within the elite itself. If the alternative is the loss of control, the elite will not resist change. More than that, the elite will accept among its members the people who challenge its traditions and, by so doing, will be in the best position to implement the new understanding of medicine.[14] Many members of the elite may continue to operate as they have in the past, and there is a need for some to do so; that is, to conduct the research which has been characteristic of the medical elite. Others, however, will concede the importance of research but will commit themselves to an understanding of medicine that emphasizes continuing and comprehensive medical care.

Many physicians predict that the new understanding of the essential purpose of medicine will be successfully implemented, and that innovations in medical education and practice will produce new training programs and delivery systems. The medical elite will persist because the future success of these innovations is apparent to its members, who will adopt what is successful so that they will continue to be accepted as the medical elite.

14. "The health and medical aspirations of the nation are largely determined outside of medicine, but it is within medicine that the means of achieving them must be created," states a report of the Citizens Commission of Graduate Medical Education.

Appendix. The Performance of Harvard Interns on Part III of the National Boards

THE NATIONAL Board of Medical Examiners made available to me a number of tests devised to measure the degree and direction of change in medical knowledge and clinical ability. In 1964, 15 Harvard interns at BCH took the Part III Examination, administered by hospital physicians under special arrangement with the National Board. Seven months later 12 of those 15 took a parallel form of the same test. The data reported here are scores of these 12. The purpose is obviously to compare performance before and after the experience of the internship.

The Part III Examination consists of three separate tests. It requires a total of 6 hours and 30 minutes to complete.

Section A (1 hour, 30 minutes) is a multiple-choice examination requiring interpretation of clinical data presented in a printed test booklet containing pictures illustrating the problems about which the questions are asked. The questions reflect the clinical and academic content of medical school.

Section B (1 hour. 30 minutes), also a multiple-choice, uses motion pictures to test acuity of observation and ability to draw proper conclusons. After watching film sequences of selected patients, the candidate is required to answer questions designed to evaluate his ability to note and interpret the observable signs.

Section C (3 hours, 30 minutes) is a programmed testing technique in which questions are answered by erasures that uncover information or report the results of actions. This section, which simulates actual clinical situations, is designed to measure clinical judgment in the management of patients. Interns were penalized for errors of omission (failure to select indicated actions) and of commission (selection of contraindicated actions).

The 1964 and 1965 scores for the 12 interns are presented in Tables A.1 and A.2. The analysis of the shift in scores is presented in Table A.2. We made no distinction between interns on the Second and Fourth Medical Services, because the total number was too small to divide. Dividing the interns into two groups would increase the chance that increments in the mean score would not be significant because of the small number of each group.

The shifts in mean scores on each of the three sections and on the entire test were determined and tested for significance. The results are presented in Table A.3. Th shift was positive throughout. For Sections A and C the shift was statistically significant at .05; for the entire test, at .01. The increment in mean score for Section B was not significant because the shifts within the group varied so greatly. The standard deviation for Section B was significantly larger than for Sections A and C.

The results indicate that the internship experience significantly increased medical knowledge and clinical competence as measured by this particular test. We discerned no significant change, however, in their ability to note and interpret observable physical signs. The individual variation in shifts on Section B indicates that this ability, as measured by the Part III Examination, depends on some unknown differences among the interns. We should note, though, that this variability can be attributed to the size of the increment in the scores of a few interns who, at the time the 1964 test was administered, had not regularly attended patients on the wards. All other interns who took the 1964 test had spent at least a few weeks on the wards regularly caring for patients. The variation therefore may stem less from individual differences in acuity than from the fact that some interns had less experience than others in taking medical histories and working up patients. The implication is that the work on the wards may add more to an ability to note and interpret physical signs than other kinds of work.

The test results also demonstrated that the performance of the 12 Harvard interns was above that of National Board candidates in general. The 1964 performance figures for the Harvard interns were obtained at the beginning of their internships; those for the National Board candidates were obtained near the end of theirs. The Harvard interns at the outset performed at least as well as other young men further along in their training.

Though interns were told that the results of the Part III Examination would be used only for my purposes, they could have thought they would be used to evaluate them personally. It is not unlikely, then, that they were highly motivated to achieve on the examination administered in 1964. The test they took in 1965 was a regular administration by the National Board of Medical Examiners. A testing effect of the kind I have described would raise a question about the implications of the fact that the mean score of the Harvard interns was above that of candidates in general. Although one could argue that the knowledge and ability of interns selected by Harvard was superior to those of medical school graduates in general, the impetus that the administration of the test as part of a research project may have had does not permit me to take that view. In other words, the high level of performance may have been as much the result of the conditions under which the test was administered as of superior medical knowledge. The Harvard interns had, as a group, an above-average knowledge of medical fact and clinical judgment. As they progressed in their training, they added to their knowledge and developed additional clinical competence.

Table A.1. The Performance of Interns on the Part III
Examination of the National Board of Medical Examiners

Intern number	Section A 1964	Section A 1965	Section B 1964	Section B 1965	Section C 1964	Section C 1965	Average 1964	Average 1965
1	88.0	92.0	88.0	92.0	89.0	84.0	88.3	89.3
2	84.0	88.0	85.0	85.0	88.0	89.0	85.7	87.3
3	91.0	95.0	90.0	94.0	90.0	96.0	90.3	95.0
4	81.0	93.0	88.0	88.0	90.0	91.0	86.3	90.7
5	90.0	86.0	86.0	87.0	85.0	94.0	87.0	89.0
6	80.0	88.0	83.0	90.0	85.0	86.0	82.7	88.0
7.	86.0	89.0	94.0	83.0	83.0	83.0	87.7	85.0
8	88.0	94.0	76.0	90.0	81.0	82.0	81.7	88.7
9	87.0	89.0	84.0	87.0	77.0	90.0	82.7	88.7
10	87.0	91.0	80.0	89.0	82.0	87.0	83.0	89.0
11	85.0	87.0	80.0	94.0	84.0	88.0	83.0	89.7
12	85.0	79.0	82.0	79.0	90.0	91.0	85.7	83.0
Mean	86.0	89.3	84.7	88.2	85.3	88.4	85.3	88.6

Table A.2. The Shift in Mean Scores on the Part III Examination
of the National Board of Medical Examiners

	1964 Mean score	1965 Mean score	Shift in scores	G.D.	Level of significance
Section A	86.0	89.3	+3.3	4.77	.05
Section B	84.7	88.2	+3.5	7.05	N.S.
Section C	85.3	88.4	+3.1	4.70	.05
Overall Part III	85.3	88.6	+3.3	3.42	.01

Index

Academia, point of contact with "real world," ix
Academic, careers in medicine, 4-5, 9-12, 59-60, 77, 237-240
medicine, 46-49, 59-60
orientation of clinical investigators, 107-108
performance by physician, 106-111, 136-137, 139-141, 143-144, 153, 231
"Academic clinic," 42, 47
Action for Boston Community Development, 40
Adjustment, in level and direction of effort by interns, 189-199
to hospital environment; see Learning
power relations during, 118-123, 127-132
Alumni, importance of, 67-68, 70, 82
American Board of Internal Medicine, 51
American Society of Clinical Investigation, 51
Anemia, pernicious, 49
Apprenticeships, 12, 231, 238
Arnstein, Margaret C., 209
Aspirations, of Harvard interns, 70-78, 86
Authority; see Power and Social exchange
Autonomy, as hallmark of physician, 92, 168, 184-185, 199-200
of medical students, 129-130
and responsibility, 81-82, 97, 181, 194

Bargaining; see Social exchange
Becker, Howard S., v, 11, 14, 32, 33, 43, 71, 82, 118, 119, 180, 189, 229
Bensman, Joseph, 125

"Bird dogs," of the medical profession, 67
Blacken, Edward, 40
Blau, Peter M., 135, 136, 138
Bloom, Samuel W., 227
Boston City Hospital, 4 et passim
brief history and description, 37, 41-42
location and patient population, 39-41
organization of, 43-46
Boston City Hospital Centennial, 38
Boston Magazine, 40
Boston, medicine in, 36
Boston Redevelopment Authority, 40
Boston, South End, 39-40
Boston Sunday Herald, 20
Brandeis University, v, 17, 20n
Brim, Orville G., 120
Bryant, W. D., 209
Bureau of Applied Social Research, 228
Bucher, Rue, 6, 8, 9, 10, 63
Byrne, John J., 37

Career, in medicine, 3-4
aspirations, 70-73
implications of internship for, 57, 59, 228-229, 240-241
lack of commitment to, 83-89, 90
ladders, 5
of Harvard physicians, 50-52, 117, 136, 148
plans, 73-78
recruitment for, 62-67, 237
requirements for, 4, 227,223-231
routes, 11-12, 60-62, 89, 125-126, 134, 241-243
"successful," 5
"symbolic," 6
Castle, William B., 37, 38, 42, 44
Citizens Commission of Graduate Medical Education, 245

Civil War, 37
Clinical investigation, 42-43, 46,
 48-49, 152, 178-179, 188-189,
 207
Clinics; see Outpatient department
Center for Community Health and
 Medical Care, vi, 88
"Cold calls," patients as, 100
Conflict, and lines of authority,
 44-45
 between interns, 205
 between interns and hospital
 administrators, 20-23
 between interns and residents,
 132, 165-166, 169-171,
 190-192
 between interns and students,
 129-130
 between interns and hospital
 employees, 21, 122-123, 156
 during field work, 19, 21, 24-25
 norms for control of, 92, 115, 123,
 131, 153-154, 159-160,
 171-172, 204-205
 within a profession, 6, 8-10
 of professional and public
 interests, 244-246
Consensus, among interns, 14-15,
 180-181, 197
Consulting physicians, 145-154
Council of Medical Education,
 Internship Review Committee
 of, 20
Cressey, Donald R., 119
Croog, Sydney H., 44

Data, analysis of, 14, 32-34, 212
 interviews, 31-32
 observation, 17-18, 24, 27-29, 209
 questionnaire, 31
 sampling, 28-29, 209-212
 special problems collecting, 19-24,
 26, 210-212
Davidson, Charles S., v
Deals; see Social exchange

Demone, Harold W., 40
Department of Health, Education
 and Welfare, vi, 50
Deutscher, Irwin, 45, 118, 232
Dowling, Harry F., 67
Drift, and career opportunities in
 medicine, 74-78, 87-88
 defaulting decisions of, 89
 process of, in medical education,
 83-87
 reasons for tolerating, 241-243

Ebert, Robert H., vi
Effort, level and direction of, 13-15,
 186, 194, 203-207, 236-238
 academic, 106-115, 190
 change in direction of, 189-202
 definition of by interns, as
 problem, 124, 130, 135, 180,
 189-190, 194, 229-230
 definition of by others, 120, 123,
 131-132, 141-144, 147, 149-
 153, 155-157, 166, 172, 188,
 190-192
 initial, 181-184
 required; see Work
Elite
 aspirations, 70-78
 careers, 11-12, 61-62, 78, 89, 116,
 134, 240
 characteristics, 47, 50-51
 and counter-elites, 8
 definition of, 5-7
 evidence for, 52-55, 61
 future of, 243-246
 medical, 9-11, 16, 30, 47, 50-52
 mission, 47-49, 117, 179
 power of, 7-9
 recruitment, 57-58, 60, 62-65,
 68-69, 239, 241-243
 training, 12-13, 178, 207, 239-241
Emergency room; see Outpatient
 department
Entry, ports of, 58-60
Eoney, James G., 244

Evans, John W., 226
Exchange; see Social exchange

Family life, of interns, 186-188
Feldman, Harvey W., 239
Field notes, 32
Field work; see Data
Finland, Maxwell, 47, 48, 53, 54, 60, 64, 65, 66, 67
Fisher, Robin A., 32
Flexner Abraham, 19
Form, W. H., 89
Freeman, Howard E., v, 44
Friedson, Eliot, 178, 226

Geer, Blanche, v, 11, 14, 33, 43, 118, 180, 229, 235
Georgopoulos, Basil, 35
Gerver, Israel, 125
Goals of interns; see Career, aspirations
Goffman, Erving, 67, 188
Goode, William J., vii, 135
Gouldner, Alvin W., 125
Graduate students, 206-207
"Great Society," the Harvard Medical Alumni Association, 67
Grand rounds, 95

Haas, Jack, 118
Hall, Oswald, 5, 35, 52
Harvard Medical Alumni Association, 67
Harvard Medical Alumni Bulletin, 48, 55, 60, 61, 65
Harvard Medical School, Department of Medicine, 37
Harvard Medical Unit: 4 *et passim*
"academic clinic," the first, 42
administration of, 44
as an elite segment of medicine, 12, 16, 47-55
as a port of entry to elite, 58-62
colonies of, 67-68

folk heroes of, 42
purposes of, 36, 117-118, 207
recruitment, policy for, 64-67, 243
Second and Fourth Medical Services of, 41
social organization of, 92, 135, 177-179
Thorndike Memorial Laboratory of, 44, 49, 136, 146
as a subculture of physicians, 36, 46, 54
at Boston City Hospital, Chapter 3
brief history and description of, 41-43
divisions of, 42-43
Homans, George C., 16
Hospital
administration of, 44-45, 115
community, 30-31, 56, 209
employees of, 155
general, 35, 223-225
objectives of, 12, 45, 91, 203
organization of, 11, 98, 177-178, 235-239
teaching and community compared, 208-226
university-affiliated, teaching, 36-37, 125, 245
House Officer's Association, 20
Hughes, Everett C., v, ix, 11, 14, 33, 43, 45, 180, 226
Hughes, Helen MacGill, 45

Infectious Disease, Division of, 39
Initial perspective, of interns, 181-185
Internal medicine, viii, 6 *passim*
Internship, 4 *et passim*
and career plans, 59, 73-74, 77-78, 83-89
and learning, 247-250
as employment, 12-13, 91
at community hospitals, 56, 208-226

"best," 81-82, 223
choice of Harvard internships, 73
criteria for judging, 78-83
experiences of, 13-14
"good," 73, 82, 223
"name," 58
purpose of, 12, 91-92, 238, 241
rotating, 56-57
specialized, 56
university-affiliated, 59
work of, Chapter 5 and Chapter 9

Jahoda, Marie, 33
Jeghers, Harold, 67
Joking, 23-25, 164-165

Kaplan, A., 7
Keefer, Chester S., 67
Kendall, Patricia, 57, 228, 235

Laboratory work, 93, 127-129, 208, 216
Lasswell, H. D., 7
Learning
    capacity for, 124
    elite, implications for, 117-118, 132-133
    initial, 118-119, 128, 135, 233-235
    a "problematic situation," 14-15, 100, 120, 180, 184, 231
    by "running around," 122-123
    to manage environment, 120, 122, 134, 184-185
    to master work, 122-123, 231
    in service organizations, 230-233, 235, 237-238
    sources of, 118, 121, 123-124, 128-129, 131-132, 162, 166, 175-176, 230-231
    ways of, 195-196
"Learning the Ropes," 118-125
Liver and Nutrition, Division of, 42
Locating equipment, 214
Long-range perspective, 15

Mann, Floyd C., 35
Mannheim, Karl, 7
Marquard, John P., 39
Matza, David, 87
Mechanic, David, 123, 206, 231, 233
Medical education, 56-57, 60, 224-228
Medical practice; see Medicine
Medical specialties, 56
Medicine
    adademic, leaders of, 49, 61
    bacteriology and pathology, era of, 48-49
    best, 152-153
    Boston, in, 36-37
    Boston City Hospital, at, 38-44, 177-178 and, particularly, Chapter 5
    celebrities of, 10-11
    changing practice of, 241
    elite of, 7-10, 121, 242
    essential purpose of, 9, 243
    "name" internships of, 58, 60, 84
    "name" schools of, 10-11, 52-55, 63, 65, 67-69, 73
    practice of, 4, 9-11, 56, 73-76, 77, 83, 89, 226
    profession, as a, 3-4, 9-11
    public, and the, 241
    subcultures of, 36, 46, 54
    training for, 56-58, 228-230, 235
    understanding of, 45-46
    understanding of, new, 244-246
    understanding of, shared by Harvard physicians, 47-48
Merton, Robert K., 6, 57, 228
Methodology; see Data
Michael Reese Hospital, 178
Miller, Andrew S., vi
Miller, Delbert, 89
Miller, George E., 229
Miller, Jessica A., vi
Miller, Roberta M., vi
Miller, Rodney J., vi

Miller, Stephen J., ix, 16, 100, 118, 120, 125, 209, 241
Mills, C. Wright, 7, 10, 50
Minot, George Richard, 42, 48, 49

National Board of Medical Examiners, 247, 249
National Intern Matching Plan, description of, 71
Night float, intern as, 98
Nurse, importance of, 120-121, 155-157, 161

Observation, participant; see Data
Office of Economic Opportunity, 244
Office of Education, vi
Outpatient department
  accident floor, 99-100, 103
  clinics at, 98
  "drop-ins," patients as, 100n, 103
  kinds of patients, 105
  opinion of, (interns), 102-104
  similarity to medical practice, 104

Parsons, Langdon, 67
Patient
  day-to-day care of, 93-97, 217-220
  interesting, 40-41, 79, 139-140, 200-201
  population, 40-41, 101-103
  typical, viii, 91, 105-106
Peabody, Francis W., 42, 49
Perspectives, 15, 180, 235
  and clinical experience, 79, 82, 195-198, 200-202
  choice of, 204
  congruence, 202-207
  initial, 181-185
  operating, 189-202
  and responsibility, 184-186, 188, 194, 199
  summarized, 186, 202
Peterson, Osler, v, 229
Power, of a professional elite, 6-8

and intellectual superiority, 8, 47
and position, 9, 49-55, 61-62
and prestige, 7, 49-50, 63
and social exchange, 123, 155-156, 165, 169, 176
of subordinates, 123, 235-236
Profession
  conceptualization of, 3, 5-11, 239-241
  elite of, 7-9, 47-55
  homogeneity of, 6, 236
  medical, 3-4, 9-11, 236
  recruitment for, 62-67, 238
  sociology of, 4-5, 62, 70, 89
Professionals
  differences between, 9
  elite, 7-8
  "successful," 5
  unanimity of, 3-4, 6

Quality, of medical education, 4, 52
Questionnaire; see Data

Rainwater, Lee, 62
Reader, George, 225
Reciprocity; see Social exchange
Recruitment, 57-58, 62-65, 68-69, 241-243
Research, medical; see Clinical investigation
Rockefeller Hospital, 49
Role models, 236
Roney, James G., Jr., 49
Rotating internship, 56
Rose, Arnold, vi, 32
Rounds
  visiting, 94-95, 112-114
  work, 93-94, 97-98
Roy, Donald, 119
"Running around," 98, 122, 214

Sanazaro, Paul, vi
Schottland, Charles, I., v
Seeman, Melvin, 229
Segments, common to professions, 9

compared to elites, 8
conditions of, Harvard Medical
    Unit, 47, 54-55
definition of, 6-7
elite, purpose of, 117
Selvin, Hanan C., 57
Service organizations, characteristics
    of, 231-233, 237-238
as training settings, 235-236
implications for training, 241-243
Shepard, William P., 49, 244
Skid Row, Boston, 40
Smith, Harvey L., 45
Social exchange, 15-16
definition of, 134-135
egalitarian relationships, 160-165,
    169, 172
interns and consulting physicians,
    145-154
interns and residents, 165-176
interns and subordinates, 155-165
interns and visiting physicians,
    138-145
and learning, 136-138
and negotiated order, 135-136,
    177-179
and power, 123, 155-156, 165,
    169, 176
and rudimentary structure, 135
rewards of, 141, 144, 151,
    153-154, 174-176
Socialization, 10
Social organization, of the Harvard
    Medical Unit, 177-179
medical profession, 5
rudimentary, 135
Sociology, of professions, 4-5, 62,
    70, 89
interactionist, 14, 16
medical education, approaches to,
    228-229
situational learning, interest in,
    119
South End, Boston, 39-40
Specialized internships, 56

Status, voluntary reduction of, 163
Stephens, William N., 33
Strauss, Anseln L., 6, 8, 9, 10, 11,
    14, 33, 43, 62 63
Succession, process of, 127-133

Teaching; see Academic,
    performance by physicians
Teaching hospital; see Hospitals
Theory, statement of, 5-9, 14-16
assumptions, 9, 17-18, 229-230
implications for analysis, 228-230
Thompson, Elizabeth J., 118, 232

Visiting rounds, 93-94, 97-98
Visiting physician, 138-145
Vona, Charles, 118

Ward management, 213-216
Wards, of the Harvard Medical
    Services, 41-42
Wagner, Thielens, Jr., 57
Wearn, Joseph T., 66
Weiss, Robert S., 125
Wheeler, Stanton, 120
Whyte, William F., 33
Wilkinson, Rupert, 240
Woods, Clyde, 118
Work, of an internship, Chapter 5
admitting patients, 96-97
emergency patient care, 98-99,
    103
experience, 91
at a general hospital, Chapter 9
off the wards, 98-106
on the wards, 92-98
patient rounds, 93-95
perspectives on, Chapter 8
realities of, 186-189
responsibility, definition of, 92
and similarity to medical practice,
    91, 104-106
and students, 111-115
Work rounds, 94-95, 112-114
Working up patients, 96, 218